Role Emerging
Occupational Ther

This book is dedicated to occupational therapists over the globe who aim to deliver services that might not match what has traditionally been delivered, or what is expected by other professionals, but always match need and promote true occupational therapy.

Role Emerging Occupational Therapy

Maximising Occupation-Focused Practice

Edited by

Miranda Thew
Mary Edwards
Sue Baptiste
and
Matthew Molineux

⬡ WILEY-BLACKWELL

A John Wiley & Sons, Ltd., Publication

This edition first published 2011 © 2011 by Blackwell Publishing Ltd

Blackwell Publishing was acquired by John Wiley & Sons in February 2007. Blackwell's publishing program has been merged with Wiley's global Scientific, Technical and Medical business to form Wiley-Blackwell.

Registered office: John Wiley & Sons Ltd, The Atrium, Southern Gate, Chichester,
West Sussex, PO19 8SQ, UK

Editorial offices: 9600 Garsington Road, Oxford, OX4 2DQ, UK
The Atrium, Southern Gate, Chichester, West Sussex, PO19 8SQ, UK
2121 State Avenue, Ames, Iowa 50014-8300, USA

For details of our global editorial offices, for customer services and for information about how to apply for permission to reuse the copyright material in this book please see our website at www.wiley.com/wiley-blackwell.

The right of the author to be identified as the author of this work has been asserted in accordance with the UK Copyright, Designs and Patents Act 1988.

Library of Congress Cataloging-in-Publication Data

Role emerging occupational therapy : maximising occupation focussed practice / edited by Miranda Thew ... [et al.].
      p. ; cm.
   Includes bibliographical references and index.
      ISBN 978-1-4051-9782-3 (pbk. : alk. paper)   1. Occupational therapy–Administration.   2. Medical care–Needs assessment.   3. Health promotion.   I. Thew, Miranda.
      [DNLM: 1. Occupational Therapy–organization & administration.   2. Community Health Services–organization & administration.   3. Health Promotion.   4. Needs Assessment.   5. Professional Role. WB 555]
      RM735.4.R65 2011
      615.8′515–dc22   2010040975

A catalogue record for this book is available from the British Library.

This book is published in the following electronic formats: ePDF 9781444339987; Wiley Online Library 9781444340006; ePub 9781444339994

Set in 10/12.5 pt Times by Aptara® Inc., New Delhi, India
Printed and bound in Malaysia by Vivar Printing Sdn Bhd

1   2011

Contents

Acknowledgements

We wish to thank the team at Wiley-Blackwell for patiently reminding us of deadlines and for their commitment to *Role Emerging Occupational Therapy*. Our inspiration for the book was from the students and professionals who have the determination to envision and deliver occupational therapy that has occupation at its heart and are willing to keep convention at bay!

Preface

"We must become the change we want to see in the world"

Mahatma Ghandi

There is an increasing push for all professionals to expand their professional boundaries and scope of practice to meet the ever-changing need within health and social care. This can pay dividends where professional roles are well recognised and where there is an established evidence-based need. In some areas within occupational therapy there has been a shrinking of the profession, in part, due to increasing genericism in the health workforce. These forces coupled with a variable job market has increased the interest in developing practice in areas that have the *potential* for occupational therapy to make a contribution, and often this is in response to changing societal demands (Rodger et al., 2007; Fortune et al., 2006). Further, some contest that unless occupational therapists grasp the move to community and away from institutionalised practice the profession will not survive (Thomas et al., 2005).

Traditional practice placement education provides occupational therapy students with important opportunities to work in settings where many of them may gain employment (Mulholland & Derdall, 2004; Rodger et al., 2007. This, in effect, prevents a break away from the medical or other such models to support expansion of the profession for the future. Where student practice placement education has taken in place in non-traditional settings there has been an increase in the awareness of occupational therapy, an occupational perspective of humans and health, and consequent employment opportunities for occupational therapists (Friedland et al., 2001; Rodger et al., 2007; Thew et al, 2008). This is surprising, given that, by definition such placements are those where there has been no previous occupational therapy role (Bossers et al., 1997) but it appears that the heightened awareness of the benefits of occupation-focused practice seems to open up opportunities for the profession.

This book focuses on the potential areas for developing occupational therapy practice and widening the impact of an occupational perspective of humans and health; it particularly offers experiences and practical examples of how an occupational perspective was introduced to a range of settings and it firmly reinforces the core and key defining skills for occupational therapists. By describing and analysing needs in settings and through addressing those needs with occupational-focused practice interventions, an occupationally focused profession is illustrated.

This book draws on the experiences of university educators, occupational therapists who have supervised or actively work in innovative settings, non-occupational therapy service providers and students who have undertaken role emerging practice placements. It provides experiential evidence underpinned by research in order to inspire and support a future vision for the profession that not only honours the uniqueness of occupational therapy, but also reflects examples of how occupation focussed intervention can address occupational injustice and meet current social and health need.

Miranda Thew, Mary Edwards, Sue Baptiste & Matthew Molineux

References

Bossers, A., Cook, J., Polatajko, H., & Laine, C. (1997). Understanding the role emerging fieldwork placement. *Canadian Journal of Occupational Therapy*, 64, 70–81.

Fortune, T., Farnworth, L., & McKinstry, C. (2006). Viewpoint: Project-focussed fieldwork: Core business or fieldwork fillers? *Australian Occupational Therapy Journal, 53* (3), 233–236.

Friedland. J., Polatajko, H., & Gage, M. (2001). Expanding the boundaries of occupational therapy practice through student field-work experiences: Description of a provisionally-funded community funded community development project. *Canadian Journal of Occupational Therapy, 68* (5) 301–307.

Mulholland, S., & Derdall, M. (2004). Bridges to Practice - Employment - Exploring what employers seek when hiring occupational therapists. *Canadian Journal of Occupational Therapy, 71* (4), 223.

Rodger, S., Thomas, Y., Dickson, D., McByrde, C., Broadbridge, J., Hawkins, R., & Edwards, A. (2007). Putting students to work: Valuing fieldwork placements as a mechanism for recruitment and shaping the future occupational therapy workforce. *Australian Occupational Therapy Journal*, 54, S94–S97.

Thew, M., Hargreaves, A., & Cronin-Davis, J. (2008). An evaluation of a role-emerging practice placement model for a full cohort of occupational therapy students. *British Journal of Occupational Therapy. 71* (8), 348–853.

Thomas, Y., Penman, M., Williamson, P. (2005). Australian and New Zealand Fieldwork: Charting territory for future practice. *Australian Occupational Therapy Journal*, 52, 78–81.

Notes on contributors

Susan Baptiste is Professor at the School of Rehabilitation Science, McMaster University, Hamilton, Ontario.

Emma Brown qualified as an occupational therapist following the MSc Occupational Therapy (pre-registration) programme at Metropolitan University. She is now working as an occupational therapist in mental health in Leeds, UK.

Lynn Cockburn is an occupational therapist and Assistant Professor at the University of Toronto, Canada.

Mary Edwards is Associate Clinical Professor at the School of Rehabilitation Science at McMaster University, Ontario, Canada.

Philippa Jane Gregory qualified as an occupational therapist following the MSc Occupational Therapy (pre-registration) programme at Metropolitan University. Philippa now resides in Singapore where she has taken a position providing Occupational Therapy for children in a private paediatric clinic.

Barbara Gurney is a Lead Cardiac Team nurse working within the Community Cardiac Services within the Leeds NHS Trust UK.

Sally Hall graduated from Leeds Metropolitan University with the MSc Occupational Therapy (pre-registration). She is an occupational therapist with a treatment service for people with mental health problems in Pontefract, West Yorkshire, UK.

Lori Letts is Associate Professor at the School of Rehabilitation Science and Assistant Dean of the Occupational Therapy Program at McMaster University, Canada.

Matthew Molineux is Associate Professor at the School of Occupational Therapy and Social Work at Curtin University, Perth, Australia.

Lydia Quelch graduated with distinction from the Leeds Metropolitan University with the MSc Occupational Therapy (pre-registration) programme and is now working as an occupational therapist within social services within the UK.

Julie Richardson is Associate Professor in the School of Rehabilitation Sciences at McMaster University, Canada.

Sylvia Rodger is Professor and Head of Division of Occupational Therapy, School of Health and Rehabilitation Sciences at The University of Queensland, Australia.

Miranda Thew is the acting programme lead of the MSc Occupational Therapy (pre-registration) programme and Principal Lecturer in Occupational Science and Occupational therapy at Leeds Metropolitan University, UK.

Yvonne Thomas is an occupational therapist and Senior Lecturer at James Cook University, Queensland, Australia.

Barry Trentham is Assistant Professor at the Department of Occupational Science and Occupational Therapy, Faculty of Medicine, University of Toronto, Canada.

Elisha Watanabe graduated from the McMaster University Occupational Therapy Program and is currently practicing as an occupational therapist in neurological and amputee rehabilitation at the Health Sciences Centre in Winnipeg, Manitoba, Canada.

Deborah Windley is Senior Lecturer in Occupational Science and Occupational therapy at Leeds Metropolitan University, UK.

Part I

Background to occupational therapy, and philosophy of occupational therapy and emergence/re-emergence of occupation-focused practice

Part One of this book is designed to open up the discussion about who we have been as occupational therapists, who we are currently and what could be the core strategies and approaches to lead us into the future, building on the essential 'fit' between academic studies and fieldwork education in the preparation of our graduates.

As most practitioners who have graduated from an occupational therapy education programme within the past two decades know, the roots of the profession were laid within the moral treatment era of the nineteenth century. Some may also know that in the mural art of Ancient Egypt were depictions of women helping others to rid themselves of foul humours through the use of activities such as playing a lyre, working on canvas and weaving on wall looms. Wherever we each believe our profession originated, one thing we all know is that somehow somewhere in the middle of the twentieth century we seemed to lose our way. In committed attempts to fit into the medical model and the reductionist thinking of the 1970s, occupational therapy relinquished its hold on occupation, and joined the movement which focused on curing, healing and ameliorating that stemmed from the perceived importance of impairment as the central construct.

One of the initiatives that has shown particular growth is the intentional strategy of integrating fieldwork education into the academic mission rather than seeing it as something that stands alone and exists in isolation at the end of study. Some settings have organised fieldwork to occur during discrete time periods such as full semesters or within a full academic year, thus creating an isolated set of experiences rather than an integrated evolution of each student working towards competence at an entry-to-practice level.

There is a distinct commitment within the current climate to create models for occupational therapy practice that are centred around 'occupation' as the core construct, using client-centred and person-centred philosophies to establish partnerships between clients and therapists. There have been steps taken to move away from settings that are formed around a medical model and a few eager pioneers who have chosen to explore new territory and not be constrained by what has been or what is; they seek to uncover what can be.

Chapter 1

Emerging occupational therapy practice: Building on the foundations and seizing the opportunities

Matthew Molineux & Sue Baptiste

Introduction

Several decades ago, Mary Reilly (1962, p. 3) proposed, perhaps quite boldly, that occupational therapy could be one of the great ideas of twentieth-century medicine. Although we might now argue about the way she located occupational therapy *within* medicine, it is probably true that many occupational therapists would agree that the sentiment of her claim was reasonable and achievable. The extent to which her prophecy has come true varies between countries, and perhaps even between different locations and organisations within countries. For example, in some countries where occupational therapy is relatively new, occupational therapists tend to work within health systems dominated by a biomedical view of humans and health, and may in some instances have their interventions directed by a medical practitioner. Even in countries where the profession is well established, some health care systems or organisations are so biomedical in their outlook that occupational therapy practice is narrowly focused and limited. However, there are also a growing number of examples of occupational therapy practice which are contemporary, innovative and effective at meeting the needs of individuals, groups and communities to achieve and maintain health through occupation, and this book provides a few examples of this work. Nonetheless, there is more work to be done by the occupational therapy profession until we can feel comfortable that Mary Reilly's challenge has been fully met.

This chapter aims to set the scene for occupational therapists and occupational therapy students as they contemplate and engage in practice which is non-traditional and so might be viewed as emerging. The chapter will begin with a brief reminder of the history of occupational therapy, with a particular focus on what constitutes contemporary occupational therapy practice. This will include the suggestion that when contemplating new and emerging practice areas focus should be shifted from a concern with what role can *occupational therapists* play in this area to a concern for what could an occupational perspective of humans and health offer. The chapter will then move on to briefly consider some of the many changes in the world, in order to begin to understand the changing nature of the practice context. The chapter will end with a section that proposes a framework for occupational therapists and occupational therapy students when contemplating developing practice in new areas.

Role Emerging Occupational Therapy: Maximising Occupation-Focused Practice, 1st edition. Edited by Miranda Thew, Mary Edwards, Sue Baptiste and Matthew Molineux. © 2011 Blackwell Publishing Ltd.

Contemporary occupational therapy

The history of occupational therapy is now very well documented with Kielhofner (2004) providing a particularly useful overview. Briefly, Kielhofner (2004) traced the history of the profession from the moral treatment movement in the eighteenth and nineteenth centuries to the current time. He showed how the profession has undergone a recurring process of paradigm–crisis–paradigm. For example, in the first 40 decades of the twentieth century the profession's paradigm was one focused on occupation. This was influenced by the core constructs of the Moral Treatment Movement and recognised, for example, that occupation was essential in human life and influenced health, and that occupation could be used to restore function lost due to disease, illness or accident. A crisis occurred when the profession was pressured by medicine to develop a more scientific basis for practice. As a result, the mechanistic paradigm emerged and so practice focused on repairing or compensating for elements of the human system that were dysfunctional or absent. When the mechanistic paradigm was recognised as not meeting the needs of people with chronic conditions or permanent impairments, another crisis ensued and resulted in the emergence of what Kielhofner (2004) has called the contemporary paradigm.

The contemporary paradigm includes a number of core constructs which at face value seem clear to occupational therapists, but which may be difficult to operationalise. The three core constructs of the contemporary paradigm are that humans have an occupational nature, the difficulties humans have in participating in occupations are the focus of occupational therapy and the defining feature of occupational therapy practice is that "engagement in occupation is the basic dynamic and core of therapy" (Kielhofner, 2004, p. 68). Although a cursory comparison of the paradigm of occupation and the contemporary paradigm might lead one to believe that there has not been much change, this would be incorrect. Indeed in some ways, this is the root of many of the problems occupational therapy faces; the "change may appear subtle, but its significance is not to be underestimated" (Molineux, 2004, p. 3).

The current paradigm reminds occupational therapists that we see the world differently from others, and therein lies our uniqueness. This is particularly important to recognise, as the world we live in is dominated by the biomedical perspective. In fact, the biomedical perspective has become so dominant, perhaps without some people realising, that it is the folk view of humans and health (Engel, 1977). Of course, the biomedical perspective is extremely useful and has been, and continues to be, of enormous benefit to humans. The advances in the diagnosis, treatment and prevention of many diseases have improved the lives of many throughout history. Wade and Halligan (2004) have usefully summarised the assumptions which are generally characteristic of a biomedical perspective:

Illness/disease is due to an underlying abnormality of the structure or function of the body
Health is the absence of disease
The patient is a passive and ideally cooperative recipient of treatment.

Although the medical field is beginning to recognise some of the problems inherent in this perspective, it continues to dominate health care systems and the professions which work within them. Of concern in the context of discussions about occupational therapy is the extent to which occupational therapists acknowledge the subtle and perhaps unrecognised influence a biomedical view of humans and health has on the development of the profession. After all, it has been recognised for some time now that the biomedical perspective is at odds with the way occupational therapists view humans and health (Rogers, 1982), and that this close alliance with medicine has been detrimental to the development of occupational therapy practice and the knowledge which underpins it (Wilcock, 1998). It is also responsible for the dilemma faced by many occupational therapists in practice, that is, being "torn between a concern to 'treat the whole person' and a concern to be credible within a medical world" that requires services to be defined within biomedical terms (Mattingly & Fleming, 1994, p. 296). Given that the outward manifestations of paradigms are inherently difficult to explicate and observe, a clear articulation of how practice might be different continues to be difficult, although there are examples in the literature.

Some might suggest that despite working within systems dominated by biomedicine it is possible to superimpose an occupational perspective. For example, Spencer et al. (1996) have provided an example of how one might overlay an occupational perspective onto a biomedical one. They suggest that following the onset of disability or illness "persons must consider which occupations they can continue to perform as they have in the past, those they can continue to perform but in new ways, and those that they may not be able to perform at all" (Spencer et al., 1996, p. 531). Although this is a useful framework and goes some way towards ensuring that an occupational perspective can be operationalised, it is nonetheless problematic. Despite recognition of changing occupational performance and engagement, the proposed framework has as its central organising construct disability and the underlying impairment. As such, it runs the risk of adopting a deficit orientation and may not recognise the way in which challenges such as illness and disability can bring positive benefits for some people and their carers (e.g. Schwartzberg, 1996; Heward et al., 2006). Nonetheless, it is one way that some occupational therapists might find useful, particularly perhaps when working in hospital environments.

The Well Elderly Study conducted by occupational therapy and occupational science researchers at the University of Southern California is an example of how an occupational perspective might be translated into practice. In this project the intervention group received a nine-month programme of individual and group sessions delivered by an occupational therapist (Clark et al., 1997; Jackson et al., 1998; Mandel et al., 1999). The participants were a group of culturally diverse older adults living in the community, and so from the start the focus was not on people with disability, but on maximising health. Furthermore, the initial modules of the programme focused on facilitating the participants to understand themselves as occupational beings and the relationship between occupational engagement and their health. Although the programme did include some techniques that might be seen as traditional occupational therapy, one of the key reasons proposed for the programme's effectiveness was that it explicitly adopted an occupational perspective (Clark et al., 2004). One simple example of this is that a module within the programme was called 'dining as an occupation'. A more traditional programme might have focused on the nutritional aspects of eating and perhaps the practicalities of cooking, including energy conservation and the use of assistive devices. In the Well Elderly Study, this module, as the title suggests, took a much broader view to include all the associated tasks and also the myriad of meanings that cooking can have for people and how these are expressed during all stages of preparing for, engaging in, finishing and reflecting on a dining experience.

In addition to the return to placing occupation at the centre of occupational therapy practice, occupational therapy and occupational science have introduced new concepts that also provide a guide to developing future practice. Occupational justice is one such concept that broadens the potential scope of occupational therapy practice, but perhaps more importantly shifts the focus away from the need and desire for occupational therapists *per se* to have a role, towards a recognition that the ideas inherent in an occupational perspective of humans and health are valuable perhaps without any direct intervention by occupational therapists.

Occupational justice was developed by Wilcock and Townsend (e.g. Wilcock & Townsend, 2000; Townsend & Wilcock, 2004) and has received much attention in the literature. Grounded on a recognition of humans as occupational beings, occupational justice is "the promotion of social and economic change to increase individual, community, and political awareness, resources, and equitable opportunities which enable people to meet their potential and experience well-being" through occupational engagement (Wilcock, 1998, p. 257). Put simply, occupational justice is concerned with creating a world in which all people have the opportunities they need to meet their needs to achieve and maintain health through occupation. Importantly, it is not about all people having the same occupational experiences. It is rather a "justice of difference that enables the prerequisites of life to be obtained according to needs, matches meaning with competence, and value with capacity and opportunity" (Wilcock, 2006, p. 247). Although this may seem a significant shift of focus for many occupational therapists, it is worth remembering that in fact the early profession was concerned with broader social issues and so this is a returning to our roots (Wood et al., 2005). Although the precise ways in which occupational justice can be translated/incorporated into practice are still being explored there are some examples (Townsend & Wilcock, 2004; Nilsson & Townsend, 2010). It is the case, however, that working in this way requires therapists to engage in broader dialogues and consider working at different levels of social systems.

In summary, currently occupational therapy finds itself within the contemporary paradigm with a growing recognition of the importance of occupational justice, and therefore must reflect on what this means for practice. A review of the underlying assumptions hint at a subtle yet significant change that brings occupation back as the central concern of occupational therapists and therefore as the organising concept for all aspects of practice. As such, it is not just a tool to be used in practice, but a whole new way of seeing the world. Indeed, it may require "a re-education into the new world view" so that occupational therapists "come to see the world with a 'new gestalt'" (Kuhn, 1970, p. 112).

The current world of health and social care

Being an occupational therapist in the twenty-first century is a challenge for a range of reasons. Although not the focus here, the pressures of daily practice are just one example of what occupational therapists must contend with, and unfortunately these may mask the bigger picture. To be an occupational therapist, and indeed any type of professional, requires a recognition of the complexity of the world within which practice occurs (Whiteford et al., 2005). More than merely recognising this complexity, however, it is necessary for occupational therapists individually and collectively to scan the practice horizon regularly to identify emerging issues that may impact on practice. This may reveal signs that a particular approach to practice might become less appropriate, as was the case when, for example, the trend in acute health care systems was for shorter hospital admissions. This required occupational therapists to review practice, as it was no longer realistic to rely on an extended period of inpatient intervention with clients before they were discharged into the community. What is more exciting are the new opportunities that might present themselves as society changes.

In order to be responsive to the changing context of practice, it is necessary to be aware of trends and developments within society. There are numerous sources of this information with each having a particular focus or perspective, and so depending on your particular interest some may be more relevant than others. Given the complexity of the issues and diversity of views, it is inappropriate to attempt to provide a comprehensive overview here. Rather, a taste of different views will be presented in an attempt to raise awareness about how important it is for occupational therapists to remain abreast of socio-cultural developments and trends.

Reporting on the most recent McKinsey global survey, Beinhocker et al. (2009) highlight a number of trends and how the recent global financial crisis has impacted on them. Although many have recognised for a long time that globalisation is a driving force in many aspects of human experience, the McKinsey survey suggests that this may not be as clear cut as previously thought. For example, it is thought that although the globalisation of goods and services will continue it is likely to stall due to the reduction in international trade, and this will also be the case for the previously mobile workforce if governments tighten immigration (Beinhocker et al., 2009). It is almost certain that boundaries will be placed on financial globalisation, given the vulnerabilities highlighted during the global financial crisis (Beinhocker et al., 2009). Related trends identified include a reducing trust in big corporations resulting in greater control and loss of flexibility of businesses, thus demanding increased government involvement in business (Beinhocker et al., 2009). Others have identified other trends to include the rise of the power of spirituality, capitalism with a conscience, consumers driven by values and the importance of social responsibility (Aburdene, 2005).

Interestingly, the Institute for the Future (2007) has documented how some of these trends might manifest at the level of individuals. For example, in the area of health and sustainability, people might use public transport more, participate in community health and well-being projects, recycle and buy recycled goods. In the health economy, people might seek out the health benefits in a range of goods and services, including food, clothing, furniture, outdoor spaces and holidays. Living a healthy lifestyle might mean having a clean home, spending time with friends and family, spending time outdoors and avoiding stress and maximising mental health. In what the Institute for the Future labels 'extended self' lies powerful insights into the beliefs people have about themselves and others. For example, personal networks might include hundreds of people spread throughout the world, people might redefine life stages as more than a chronology, and that people need to process larger amounts of information more quickly in order to interact effectively. Although only a taste of what *might* be, these few examples open up a number of opportunities for using an occupational perspective to support people in these new ways of living.

From this cursory overview of just a few sources and merely from living in the world ourselves, it is clear that both the pace and magnitude of change are great. Although we should continue to be aware of what futurists and others (in fields well beyond occupational therapy and health care) have to say about our changing world, as a profession occupational therapy must be clear about what it has to offer the society and to explore frameworks to guide the development of the profession and the practice of individuals to ensure it can meet the ever-changing needs of individuals, groups and communities.

Bringing it together

People respond to change in different ways, and so for some the changes in the world, and health and social care may appear daunting. However, these changes offer huge potential for occupational therapy to break out of the confines of traditional health and social care and finally be one of the world's great ideas and so rise to the challenge set by Reilly (1962). In order to move towards this future it is necessary for occupational therapists to recognise that they are members of a profession, and to reflect on what that means. A profession is a group "recognised by society as having expertise in assisting people in resolving specific practical problems" (Mosey, 1996, p. 10). In this, it is implicit that the practice of the profession is based on largely intellectual operations for which the individual professional has responsibility, practice is based on science and learning and has a practical and definite end that is of benefit to society (Flexner, 2001).

What then is the focus of occupational therapy's contribution to society? Although all occupational therapists could no doubt describe the fine detail of their practice, it is noteworthy that apart from the work of the Canadian Association of Occupational Therapists over the years (Canadian Association of Occupational Therapists, 1991; Townsend & Polatajko, 2007) there is no "simple generic occupational therapy philosophical statement that everyone in the profession learns and uses" (Wilcock, 2000, p. 82). This means that at times the profession may appear fragmented and disjointed and this has been accentuated over the years as therapists move into increasingly specialised areas of practice. Although some may argue this is not a problem for practitioners in more traditional settings (although many of those practitioners will recognise it is a problem for them as well), this situation is particularly problematic when it comes to exploring new and emerging areas of practice. For example, how would an occupational therapist determine the scope and boundaries of practice in a novel practice area?

Fortune (2000) explored this in her study exploring the extent to which occupational therapy practice in child and adolescent mental health was occupation focused. One part of her interviews with occupational therapists included asking them to respond to a hypothetical scenario about what they might offer if working in a community youth centre. One of the findings from the study was that for some participants their response to this hypothetical scenario was "devoid of a philosophical reference to occupation" (Fortune, 2000, p. 227). These therapists suggested that their contribution to the team would be dependent on their colleagues, their clients and the practice context. This study provides a powerful example of the problems (Wilcock, 1999) identified by occupational therapy not having a professional philosophy.

In her paper, Wilcock (1999) highlighted that occupational therapy did not have a shared professional philosophy and that this caused three problems. First, without a philosophy it is not possible to identify the core skills required to practice occupational therapy and what are peripheral, or perhaps even inappropriate, skills and techniques for occupational therapist to employ. Second, because of a lack of shared understanding of the boundaries of practice, what occupational therapists do and the way they describe their practice tends to be quite concrete and focused at the impairment level. Because of this it could be difficult to see how a therapist working with someone following a hand injury is similar to another therapist working with someone who is a refugee. Although the practicalities of therapy might be very different, use of a common language arising from a professional philosophy would enable the shared focus on achieving and maintaining health through occupation to be recognised. Third, without a professional philosophy the future development of the profession runs the risk of being ad hoc, disjointed and lacking in coherence. All these problems mean that working in new and emerging areas in response to a changing world and the emerging needs of individuals, groups and communities can seem daunting. Wilcock (1999) suggested, not surprisingly, that the philosophy of occupational therapy should be one of *occupation for health*. She also provided a framework which can be used to consider what contribution an occupational perspective of humans and health can offer in any setting.

In the first edition of her seminal work *An Occupational Perspective of Health*, Wilcock (1998) proposed two triangles to understand the occupational factors that lead to health/well-being and ill health. The triangles demonstrate how disease, disability and death (Figure 1.1) and health and well-being (Figure 1.2) can be understood by exploring the underlying occupational influences. The strength of these frameworks is that they make it possible to move beyond the level of the individual person (the second highest level on each triangle) to consider the range of institutions and factors which act to influence an individual's state of health or ill health. Viewing health issues in this way, occupational therapists can, perhaps for the first time, begin to consider the ways legislation, fiscal policies, the media, and the structure of health and education systems influence occupational engagement and therefore health. Further still, they bring attention to the way underlying occupational factors such as the type of economy, national policies and priorities, and cultural values give rise to particular occupational institutions that then shape occupational engagement.

Many occupational therapists continue to be located within health and social care systems and so mostly only work with people once they are experiencing a health disorder (the second highest level in Figure 1.1). Using Wilcock's triangles, therapists in these situations can reflect on their clients' experiences and contexts to gain a deeper understanding of the forces which have led the client to require support from health and social services. As such, it can only strengthen the therapist's ability to work in a client-centred way and thereby maximise the beneficial outcome of the therapeutic partnership.

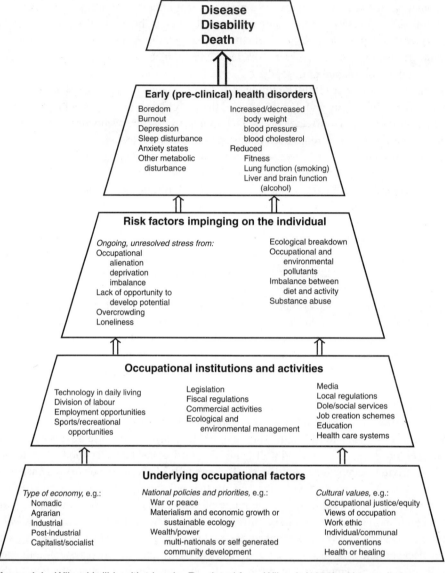

Figure 1.1   Wilcock's ill-health triangle. Reprinted from Wilcock (1998) with permission.

More exciting, however, is how seeing health in this way opens up a myriad of new opportunities for occupational therapists to influence the health of not only individuals but whole communities, regions and even countries. For example, imagine the impact an occupational therapist could have by working with, or even within, popular media to shape the messages conveyed through advertising. The result might be an advertising campaign which sends the message of the health benefits of occupational engagement. It might also mean a change to advertising and broadcasting standards to ensure that diversity is represented more often and more positively, so that prevailing stereotypes are

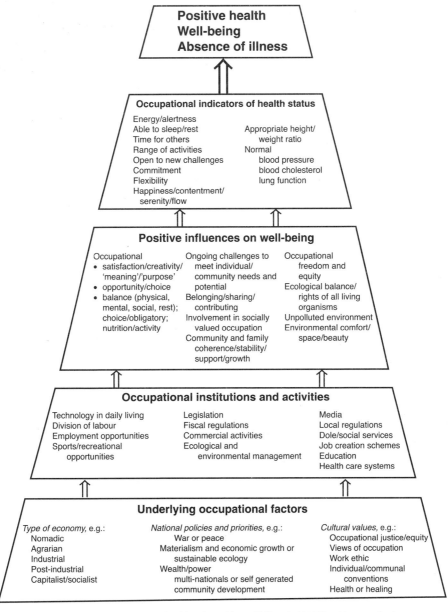

Figure 1.2   Wilcock's health triangle. Reprinted from Wilcock (1998) with permission.

challenged and stigma reduced. Similarly, in countries with financial benefit programmes for people who are unemployed what might an occupational perspective bring? People with low incomes are at risk of occupational deprivation due to the costs associated with many occupations in capitalist societies, and so an occupational perspective might lead to an increase in benefits, a greater range of free or discounted occupational opportunities, or more occupationally orientated vocational training and support programmes.

The power of an occupational perspective in addressing the broader social issues facing the world has been recognised within occupational therapy, but the focus on ill health and the limits of a biomedical perspective have restricted the profession developing into non-traditional areas. This has begun to change. For example, several books provide many examples of how adopting an occupational perspective can open up opportunities for enhancing health through occupation (Kronenberg et al., 2004; Pollard et al., 2008). Similarly there is a small, but growing amount of research which explores and documents the impact of an occupational perspective with a wider range of individuals such as young people at risk of gang involvement (Snyder et al., 1998) and older people living independently in the community (Jackson et al., 1998; Mountain et al., 2008). More recently, a special issue of the *American Journal of Occupational Therapy* focused on social justice and health disparities and demonstrated a range of innovative ways an occupational perspective can be applied. For example, in their paper Blakeney and Marshall (2009) examined water quality. Although the occupational implications of water quality might not be immediately apparent, this study showed that poor water quality resulted in residents experiencing occupational imbalance, occupational deprivation and occupational alienation. Research such as this opens the doors for contributing an occupational perspective towards work on achieving the United Nations's (2008) Millennium Development Goals, which includes access to safe drinking water within the targets of one goal.

Ultimately, unless the profession of occupational therapy takes a stance on viewing changes in the world and the impact of these on health and well-being, occupational therapy will continue to follow studiously in the shadow of the other professions. If this is the case then the promise of occupational therapy will not be realised. Through articulating, implementing and sharing the unique occupational perspective with the aim of achieving occupational justice the profession can contribute positively to society.

Conclusion

This chapter has provided a broad overview of occupational therapy in the context of the changing world that the profession and individual occupational therapists exist within. For many years now, and for many more to come, occupational therapy will be influenced by a whole range of social, cultural, political and financial pressures (just to name a few). Although some may see this ever-changing world as threatening, it needs to be recast as a time of great possibility. Although there are, without doubt, some very real threats to the profession and the potential contribution it can make, we must turn to our unique professional perspective for security. It is only by engaging with an occupational perspective of humans and health, and then translating that into the vast array of practice opportunities that are out there can we meet the challenge set by one of the profession's leaders. To paraphrase Reilly (1962), occupational therapy *must* be one of the great ideas of the twenty-first century. It is our professional responsibility to make sure it is, simply because there are so many individuals, groups and communities who experience occupational injustice, and so many more who are at risk.

References

Aburdene, P. (2005). *Megatrends 2010: The Rise of Conscious Capitalism*. Newburyport: Hampton Roads Publishing.

Beinhocker, E., Davis, I., & Mendonca, L. (2009). The 10 trends you have to watch. *Harvard Business Review*, *87* (7/8), 55–60.

Blakeney, A. B., & Marshall, A. (2009). Water quality, health, and human occupations. *American Journal of Occupational Therapy*, *63* (1), 46–57.

Canadian Association of Occupational Therapists. (1991). *Occupational Therapy Guidelines for Client-Centered Practice*. Toronto: CAOT Publications.

Clark, F., Azen, S., Zemke, R., Jackson, J., Carlson, M., Mandel, D., Hay, J., Josephson, K., Cherry, B., Hessel, C., Palmer, J., & Lipson, L. (1997). Occupational therapy for independent-living older adults. *Journal of the American Medical Association*, *278* (16), 1321–1326.

Clark, F., Jackson, J., & Carlson, M. (2004). Occupational science, occupational therapy and evidence based practice: What the Well Elderly Study has taught us. In M. Molineux (Ed.), *Occupation for Occupational Therapists* (pp. 200–218). Oxford: Blackwell Publishing.

Engel, G. (1977). The need for a new medical model: A challenge for biomedicine. *Science*, *196* (4286), 129–136.

Flexner, A. (2001). Is social work a profession? *Research on Social Work Practice*, *11* (2), 152–165.

Fortune, T. (2000). Occupational therapists: Is our therapy truly occupational or are we merely filling gaps? *British Journal of Occupational Therapy*, *63* (5), 225–230.

Heward, K., Molineux, M., & Gough, B. (2006). A grounded theory analysis of the occupational impact of caring for a partner who has multiple sclerosis. *Journal of Occupational Science*, *13* (3), 188–197.

Institute for the Future. (2007). *2006 Ten-year Forecast Signals Survey*. Palo Alto: Institute for the Future.

Jackson, J., Carlson, M., Mandel, D., Zemke, R., & Clark, F. (1998). Occupation in lifestyle redesign: The well elderly study occupational therapy programme. *American Journal of Occupational Therapy*, *52* (5), 326–336.

Kielhofner, G. (2004). *Conceptual Foundations of Occupational Therapy* (3rd ed.). Philadelphia: F.A. Davis.

Kronenberg, F., Algado, S., & Pollard, N. (Eds.). (2004). *Occupational Therapy Without Borders: Learning From The Spirit of Survivors*. Edinburgh: Churchill Livingstone.

Kuhn, T. (1970). *The Structure of Scientific Revolutions* (2nd ed.). Chicago: University of Chicago Press.

Mandel, D., Jackson, J., Zemke, R., Nelson, L., & Clark, F. (1999). *Lifestyle Redesign: Implementing the Well Elderly Program*. Bethesda: American Occupational Therapy Association.

Mattingly, C., & Fleming, M. (1994). *Clinical Reasoning: Forms of Inquiry in a Therapeutic Practice*. Philadelphia: F.A. Davis.

Molineux, M. (2004). Occupation in occupational therapy: A labour in vain? In M. Molineux (Ed.), *Occupation for Occupational Therapists* (pp. 1–14). Oxford: Blackwell Publishing.

Mosey, A. C. (1996). *Applied Scientific Inquiry in the Health Professions: An Epistemological Orientation* (2nd ed.). Bethesda: American Occupational Therapy Association.

Mountain, G., Mozley, C., Craig, C., & Ball, L. (2008). Occupational therapy led health promotion for older people: Feasibility of the Lifestyle Matters programme. *British Journal of Occupational Therapy*, *71* (10), 406–413.

Nilsson, I., & Townsend, E. (2010). Occupational justice – Bridging theory and practice. *Scandinavian Journal of Occupational Therapy*, *17* (1), 57–63.

Pollard, N., Sakellariou, D., & Kronenberg, F. (Eds.). (2008). *A Political Practice of Occupational Therapy*. Edinburgh: Churchill Livingstone Elsevier.

Reilly, M. (1962). Occupational therapy can be one of the great ideas of 20th Century medicine. *American Journal of Occupational Therapy, 16* (1), 1–9.

Rogers, J. (1982). Order and disorder in medicine and occupational therapy. *American Journal of Occupational Therapy, 36* (1), 29–35.

Schwartzberg, S. (1996). *A Crisis of Meaning: How Gay Men are Making Sense of AIDS*. New York: Oxford University Press.

Snyder, C., Clark, F., Masunaka-Noriega, M., & Young, B. (1998). Los Angeles street kids: New occupations for life program. *Journal of Occupational Science, 5* (3), 133–139.

Spencer, J., Davidson, H., & White, V. (1996). Continuity and change: Past experience as adaptive repertoire in occupational adaptation. *American Journal of Occupational Therapy, 50* (7), 526–534.

Townsend, E., & Polatajko, H. (Eds.). (2007). *Enabling Occupation II: Advancing an Occupational Therapy Vision for Health, Well-being, & Justice Through Occupation*. Ottawa: Canadian Association of Occupational Therapists.

Townsend, E., & Wilcock, A. (2004). Occupational justice and client-centred practice: A dialogue in progress. *Canadian Journal of Occupational Therapy, 71* (2), 75–87.

United Nations. (2008). Millennium Development Goals – Goal 7: Esnure environmental sustainability. Retrieved 15 May 2010, from http://www.un.org/millenniumgoals/environ.shtml.

Wade, D., & Halligan, P. (2004). Do biomedical models of illness make for good healthcare systems? *British Medical Journal, 329* (7479), 1398–1401.

Whiteford, G., Klomp, N., & Wright-St Clair, V. (2005). Complexity theory: Understanding occupation, practice and context. In G. Whiteford & V. Wright-St Clair (Eds.), *Occupation and Practice in Context* (pp. 3–15). Sydney: Churchill Livingstone.

Wilcock, A. (1998). *An Occupational Perspective of Health*. Thorofare: Slack.

Wilcock, A. (1999). The Doris Sym Memorial Lecture: Developing a philosophy of occupation for health. *British Journal of Occupational Therapy, 62* (5), 192–198.

Wilcock, A. (2000). Development of a personal, professional and educational occupational philosophy: An Australian perspective. *Occupational Therapy International, 7* (2), 79–86.

Wilcock, A. (2006). *An Occupational Perspective of Health* (2nd ed.). Thorofare: Slack.

Wilcock, A., & Townsend, E. (2000). Occupational justice. *Journal of Occupational Science, 7*, 84–86.

Wood, W., Hooper, B., & Womack, J. (2005). Reflections on occupational justice as a subtext of occupation-centred education. In F. Kronenberg, S. Algado & N. Pollard (Eds.), *Occupational Therapy Without Borders: Learning from the Spirit of Survivors* (pp. 378–389). Edinburgh: Elsevier.

Chapter 2

Models of role emerging placements

Mary Edwards & Miranda Thew

Introduction

As the previous section has highlighted, education of any health and social care professional has to match contemporary national and international political drivers. These can be related to the technological advancement of medicine; the movement towards rehabilitation into local communities, relying on informal carers and non-statutory organisations and the ever-increasing role that health promotion is playing particularly in primary care. Role emerging placements can be useful in helping students to understand how occupational therapy practice can meet these contemporary challenges and changes. Role emerging placements usually occur in settings that have previously not had an occupational therapist in post. The student considers the needs of the setting in terms of occupational therapy and either establishes an occupational therapy role, or carries out a project which demonstrates an occupational perspective that may benefit the placement setting or service users.

The World Federation of Occupational Therapists (2002) standards for fieldwork education advocate innovative placements such as those taking place in settings lacking occupational therapy provision. Studies suggest that role emerging placements are an important element of occupational therapy practice and that they promote and increase the awareness of the profession with a corresponding demand for services (Friedland et al., 2001; Thomas et al., 2005). Research also suggests that students are more independent and autonomous following experience in a role emerging placement, resulting in increased professional growth and development of life-long learning abilities (Alsop & Donald, 1996; Bossers et al., 1997). When role emerging placements have been compared to placement in more traditional settings, the role emerging placement has developed to be at least an equivalent, but sometimes a superior, learning experience for students (Friedland et al., 2001; Thew et al., 2008). Students have highlighted that the value of these placements is that they offer opportunities to promote the profession and develop a professional identity (Bossers et al., 1997; Huddleston, 1999).

This chapter describes and discusses the shared and contrasting features of two examples of role emerging placement models for occupational therapy pre-registration students.

Role Emerging Occupational Therapy: Maximising Occupation-Focused Practice, 1st edition. Edited by Miranda Thew, Mary Edwards, Sue Baptiste and Matthew Molineux. © 2011 Blackwell Publishing Ltd.

This includes how to prepare supervisors and students, with clarification of the roles and responsibilities of all involved; how to establish, facilitate and integrate the placement within the curriculum; examples of the kinds of settings that students have attended on placement are offered, and finally the lessons learnt by academic staff are discussed and explored in establishing such placements. The two differing models described are based in two pre-registration occupational therapy curricula on two international continents, namely, at Leeds Metropolitan University in the United Kingdom (UK) and McMaster University in Ontario, Canada. The conclusion offers suggestions and recommendations for academic staff, occupational therapists and students in how to get the most out of such a potentially rich, rewarding yet challenging learning experience.

The practice placement situation in Canada and the UK

Many university occupational therapy programmes in Canada are involved in offering role emerging practice (REP) placements and have done so for several years (Jung et al., 2005). Models to establish, develop and evaluate these experiences vary across programmes. Student roles can include but are not limited to conducting needs assessment, direct clinical service, programme development, consultation and community development. Role emerging placements for students in the UK were encouraged by the College of Occupational Therapists (COT) (2006) to expand placement opportunities partly in response to a shortage of suitable placements (Fisher & Savin-Baden, 2002; Casares et al., 2003). It now appears that such a placement within the pre-registration occupational therapy curricula is becoming the norm (Wood, 2005; Fieldhouse & Fadden, 2009). Increasingly, students and educators are recognising the benefits rather than the deficiencies of such placements (Lloyd et al., 2002; Overton, et al., 2009; Wilcock et al., 2009). However, the vast majority of academic institutions appear to offer these settings as elective placements for a minority of students (Wood, 2005).

The College of Occupational Therapists (2006) has developed guidance for such practice placements, and recently there has been an increasing amount of evidence to support such placements within the UK (Hook & Kenny, 2007; Martin & Daniels, 2007; Thew et al., 2008; Fieldhouse & Fadden, 2009). However, there appears to be anxiety associated with students feeling apprehensive regarding expectations of the settings and the university (Mitchell & Kampfe 1990 in Spiliotopoulou, 2007; Mulholland & Derdall, 2005; Thew et al, 2008). There is also some concerns that the non-traditional settings for students could put the students at risk of being 'exploited' as an extra pair of hands and/or that clients would be left 'high and dry' with a service being offered and then withdrawn at the end of the placement (Wood, 2005). Others have suggested that students need to meet a certain criteria in order to be considered suitable for such a placement (Jepson et al., 2007). The ultimate issue here is that the UK, like Canada and Australia, consider the non-traditional or emerging role placement to be 'riskier' than the more traditional NHS/Social Services route where the occupational therapy supervision is 'in-house' (Prigg & Mackensie, 2002). Risk may be in terms of the student not being taught specific occupational therapy techniques and skills and in not receiving adequate support (Friedland et al., 2001; Prigg & Mackensie, 2002). Nevertheless, the programme at Leeds Metropolitan University has demonstrated that it is feasible to provide a role emerging placement to more than just an elective few, and that it can be an expectation for *all* occupational therapy pre-registration students (Thew et al., 2008). That said, the cohort is relatively small (currently only 18), therefore cannot be comparable to the more usual, larger, cohort size. It is considered by many students to be a superior learning experience to that of a traditional practice placement, regarding understanding and demonstrating the value of occupation focused interventions and philosophy (Thew et al, 2008), although more research regarding the relative benefits of such placements is clearly required (Overton et al., 2009).

Models of Role Emerging placements in Canada and the UK

McMaster University, Ontario, Canada

The McMaster University occupational therapy programme is a two-year professional Master's entry level to practice programme. There is a cohort of 60 to 65 students in each year. There are five practice placements throughout the two-year programme; three in first year, and two in the second year. These practice placements are designed to provide the students with the opportunity to apply and build upon their knowledge, skills and behaviours in a range of practice settings, with clients of various ages facing a diversity of occupational issues. At McMaster, it is not mandatory for each student to engage in an REP setting. These practice sites are constantly being developed and, at present, approximately one third of the class has the opportunity to participate in an REP placement. Each academic term where role emerging placements are offered includes a practice placement period of six or eight weeks. In order that the students have a reasonable grounding in occupational therapy theory, role and scope of practice, REP experiences are offered mainly in the second year of the programme. In some instances, when sufficient numbers of 'traditional' placements are not available, students have engaged in REP settings at the end of the first year. When this occurs, care must be taken to ensure that the student is mature enough to deal with the experience and adequate support is provided. Students are assigned to role emerging practice settings in pairs in order to benefit from a collaborative learning model (DeClute & Ladyshewsky, 1993).

Identification and preparation of practice placement sites

Over the years, opportunities for REP sites have been identified in various ways. Faculty involvement in community development initiatives or membership on community boards has identified new potential partnerships for learning. Students may identify a clinical interest that they wish to pursue, or an individual or organisation may contact the university to request the development of a learning partnership. Non-occupational therapy service providers in various organisations have also identified the need to explore the potential contributions that an occupational therapy perspective could add to their current services. More recently, government-funded research projects focusing on rehabilitation in primary care or community development have also resulted in REP-learning opportunities for students. A list of settings/sites utilised for REP at McMaster is found in Table 2.1.

Table 2.1   Settings for role emerging placements – McMaster University.

Setting	Focus for role emerging practice
Alzheimer Society of Niagara Region	Community programme for persons with dementia and their caregivers
Brain Injury Services of Hamilton	Residential and community integration programme for persons with acquired brain injury
Peel Halton Acquired Brain Injury Services	Residential and community integration programme for persons with acquired brain injury
Camp Robin Hood	Summer camp for able bodied children and children with disabilities
Canadian National Institute for the Blind	Direct and consultation for low vision; complex health issues including low vision
Claremont House	Harm Reduction programme for homeless individuals with addiction
Community Living, Hamilton	Residential and workshop setting for persons with developmental delay
Express Yourself	Private programme for children with speech delay and associated developmental issues
Halton Catholic District School Board	Consultation with Special Education Teams and direct work with children with special needs; elementary and secondary
Halton District School Board – Woodview School	Public school programme for children with mental health and behavioural issues
Hamilton Health Sciences Corporation – Eating Disorders Clinic – in exploration	Direct service and consultation – persons with eating disorders; mental health
Lions Foundation of Canada – Special Skills Dogs of Canada	Specialised training programme for individuals receiving special service dogs (for visual loss, hearing loss and general service requirements)
North Hamilton Community Health Centre	Primary care community health centre
McMaster Family Practice Unit	Primary care community health centre
McMaster University Employee Work life Support Services	University: return to work, job site analysis
(The) Paddle Programme (North Bay, North East Ontario)	Adolescents and adults with developmental disabilities in community
Rygiel Supports for Community Living	Residential and community integration services for individuals with developmental delay and multiple disabilities
Paradigm Rehabilitation and Nursing Services	Residential and community integration programme for persons with acquired brain injury
PATH Employment Services – in exploration	Vocational issues with persons with disabilities
School of Rehabilitation Science- Accessibility Audit	Campus audit and education re-access issues (physical, social)

Table 2.1 Settings for role emerging placements – McMaster University. (*Continued*)

Setting	Focus for role emerging practice
Shelter Health Network	Community/marginalised groups
Settlement Integration Services Organization – pending	Consultation and direct work with newly immigrated persons
Six Nations of the Grand River Reserve	First Nations setting – primary care and preschool screening programme
McMaster University Sport Fitness School	Consultation and direct with children with special needs
Stonechurch Family Practice Unit	Primary care
TALC Academy	Private programme for children with speech delay and associated developmental issues
YWCA	Community services for homeless

Following these student placements, some settings have identified the need for ongoing occupational therapy involvement and this has resulted in an occupational therapist position being established. Other settings may identify the need for occupational therapy service but have been unable to establish a budgeted position to meet those needs.

Once a potential opportunity for a role emerging placement is identified, the university Professional Practice Coordinator (PPC) contacts the individual/facility/agency to more fully explore the value/possibility of developing a learning partnership. This usually involves an initial telephone conversation to begin to clarify expectations and outline the requirements that must be met from both the university and agency perspectives. If this results in a continued interest to further develop the relationship, a site visit is arranged for the PPC to see the potential practice setting, meet the relevant agency participants and continue the dialogue to ensure that the partnership is a win-win situation while meeting the educational requirements of the university. The needs of the setting and potential student roles/projects are discussed. It is important to clearly state that this is a learning opportunity for both the students and the agency/setting. All must be aware that the students will be actively examining how an occupational therapist can augment and complement existing services provided in the setting and they will not merely be additional resources to help carry out existing services. Each member of the partnership must have an open view of current programming/service provision and be prepared to consider and reflect on potential changes to enhance the client experience. Expectations for adequate supervision of students and the evaluation of student performance are also reviewed and plans to address the requirements are made.

Supervision during the placement

Since there is no occupational therapist on site in an REP setting, it is necessary to identify an on-site contact for the students. This individual will facilitate the students' understanding of the service/agency and facilitate processes such as initial orientation and needs assessment, client referrals and programme development. If the setting is used repeatedly for student learning opportunities, the on-site contact can be a resource for the development of legacy resource materials such as procedure manuals, information on relevant community resources, samples of assessment forms or documentation to help ensure that subsequent students are able to build on the experience of previous learners. The need for and identification of an occupational therapist (off-site) to provide discipline-specific guidance and student evaluation is also key to the development of a viable learning partnership and to meet both professional college (College of Occupational Therapist of Ontario, 1996) and university educational requirements. Off-Site occupational therapy supervisors must agree to be available remotely (by phone or email) throughout the work week and commit to being on site a minimum of 1 day per week throughout the placement period. This will allow for both direct and indirect involvement in teaching, learning, feedback and formal evaluation. Since this is a significant commitment for the off-site (occupational therapy) supervisor, an honorarium to acknowledge these contributions has been established. This honorarium is not equivalent to a standard salary, but is augmented by various benefits available through the university such as access to electronic library services and preceptor educational events. Box 2.1 outlines the roles and responsibilities for students, on site and off site supervisors and the PPC.

Selection and preparation of students

Student allocation to REP settings is determined through discussion with the PPC who is responsible for ensuring that all students have a variety of clinical learning experiences. Students may self-identify the desire to engage in a particular practice area, and, on occasion, students have identified new settings for role emerging placement development. Students may identify a particular interest in REP as a result of discussions with practicing clinicians in previous clinical placements, following an academic assignment that may have inspired them to consider new or different occupational therapy roles or practice areas, or as a result of personal experience in the health care system, for example, the identification of frustrating gaps in current service or the potential for expanded roles for occupational therapy. Alternatively, a list of potential REP settings is presented to the students who then indicate their preferences for placement locations.

Prior to the commencement of the placement, a meeting is arranged with the students, the on-site (non-occupational therapist) supervisor, the occupational therapy off-site supervisor and the PPC. This is preferably held at the practice location to enable the students to see the physical surroundings in which they will be learning, meet key agency individuals and supervisors, and become aware of potential resources available and to ensure a common understanding of the expectations of the learning experience. Clarification of methods to ensure clear and consistent communication (e.g. how best to contact supervisors in both routine and emergency situations) is also critical at this point in the development of the educational partnership. This meeting can be instrumental in reducing student anxiety related to the 'unknown' nature of the learning experiences and can help establish a positive working relationship between all parties involved.

Box 2.1   Roles and responsibilities within the REP at McMaster

Student Roles and Responsibilities

In any and all placement experiences, student occupational therapists are expected to actively participate in assigned practice to acquire and/or apply knowledge, therapeutic skills and clinical reasoning skills pertaining to the setting. Students are expected to participate in planned learning activities and engage in self-directed learning and open communication in order to meet the practicum expectations and standards. This is also true in role emerging placements.

The responsibilities of the students in all placements are as follows:

1. To follow all policies and procedures of the facility, including those regarding dress and general conduct
2. To take responsibility for his or her own learning
3. To develop and implement learning objectives (including resources, evidence and validation) as components of the Competency Based Fieldwork Evaluation for Occupational Therapists (CBFE-OT). The CBFE-occupational therapist serves as the basis for learning and for evaluation of student performance
4. To prepare a written self-evaluation at Midterm and Final, for review with Preceptor
5. To actively participate in experiential learning and maximise opportunities for client involvement
6. To work collaboratively with other health care professionals and caregivers to deliver quality service
7. To accept and respond appropriately to feedback, and to provide feedback to the preceptor and other team members as appropriate
8. To communicate with the Professional Practice Coordinator regarding any problems or other issues related to the practicum experiences
9. To support the MSc(OT) Programme philosophy and goals, and to act as an effective representative of the programme
10. To demonstrate professional behaviour that is consistent with the College of Occupational Therapists of Ontario (COTO) Code of Ethics, Guidelines for Professional Behaviours in Clinical Encounters, and COTO Essential Competencies of Practice for Occupational Therapists, 2nd edition, June 2003
11. To follow the principles and guidance of *Enabling occupation II: Advancing an occupational therapy vision for health, well-being, & justice through occupation* (Townsend & Polatajko, 2007) as a basis for client evaluation and intervention
12. To disclose and manage in a timely way any limitations that may affect their ability to do the essential components of clinical activity or put other staff or patients/clients at risk

In addition to the aforementioned responsibilities students are also expected to:

1. review role emerging fieldwork practice handbook prior to the start of the placement
2. review any information provided by the facility and meet with the professional practice coordinator and offsite preceptor prior to the start of the placement
3. send the introductory practicum letter to both the offsite preceptor and the onsite supervisor
4. research the fieldwork placement site and if possible, contact students who have previously had a placement at the facility to learn more and to establish a potential peer support

Due to the self-directed learning skills required it is the expectation that students will be at a level 2 or above on the McMaster University Occupational Therapy Professional Practice Experiences & Fieldwork Levels (see addendum page). In a role emerging fieldwork placement, the onus is on the student(s) to be self-directed, organised and to manage learning opportunities and evaluation.

(Continued)

Box 1.1   (*Continued*)

Offsite (occupational therapist) Preceptor Roles & Responsibilities

Consistent with all other types of placements, offsite, role emerging preceptors will have a minimum of one year professional experience and hold credentials with the appropriate regulatory body.

The role of the offsite preceptor is

1. to support the student's learning about occupation, occupational performance, occupational engagement and how to address those concepts with clients in a setting in which there is not currently an established occupational therapy role or programme
2. to provide ongoing supervision throughout the practicum; however, the offsite preceptor will communicate and develop with the student the preferred methods of communication throughout the placement and the frequency regarding attendance at the facility for onsite preceptorship
3. to develop and maintain skills as a preceptor through continuing education e.g. attendance at workshops and seminars;
4. to support and understand the MSc(OT) Programme philosophy and goals and be aware of curriculum content, professional preparation objectives and evaluation strategies;
5. to provide the opportunity for the student to participate in appropriate learning situations in order that the student is able to meet personal and programme objectives;
6. to create a climate in which the student can practice self-appraisal;
7. to create a climate in which the student can be open to give and receive feedback;
8. to provide feedback to the student in a meaningful and timely way: Verbal feedback throughout placement; written and verbal at Midterm and Final Evaluations
9. to facilitate and encourage self-directed learning in the student;
10. to function both as a resource and process consultant to the student;
11. to assist the student in developing learning objectives (including resources, evidence & validation) as components of the CBFE-OT particular to the setting, client population and needs of the student;
12. to evaluate student performance based on the objectives and evaluation criteria outlined in the CBFE-OT;
13. to submit documentation regarding student performance and to <u>recommend</u> a final evaluation to Professional Practice Coordinator;
14. to communicate with the Professional Practice Coordinator (as needed) re: expectations of students and evaluation of performance.

Onsite Supervisor Roles and Responsibilities

The onsite supervisorhas the following roles:
1. To provide orientation to the facility/setting/programme including:
   - a physical tour of the facility and student "work area" (e.g. Student work space, location for student to receive mail and/or correspondence, lunch area, etc)
   - a review of the organisational structure and culture of the facility
   - the rules and regulations within the facility the student is to adhere to
   - introduction of the student(s) to other staff members at the site
   - training or arranging for training for students on any needed computer programs, technology or equipment that is required
   - identification of onsite resources that may be of benefit to the student
   - emergency procedures.
2. To communicate with the offsite preceptor and/or professional practice coordinator to share feedback regarding student performance.

(Continued)

Box 1.1   (*Continued*)

Professional Practice Coordinator Roles and Responsibilities

In all practicum experiences, the role of the Professional Practice Coordinator is to develop and manage the professional preparation component of the curriculum. The Coordinator acts as a resource to *both* the student and preceptor. In role emerging placements, the coordinator acts as a resource for the student, offsite preceptor and onsite supervisor at the placement facility.

The Professional Practice Coordinator in role emerging placements has the following roles:

1. To ensure a process exists for approving sites: review, monitor and evaluate sites, review and revise the professional practice and role emerging handbooks on an annual basis; and organise and conduct educational workshops for offsite preceptors and onsite supervisors.
2. To negotiate with facility-based coordinators the number of students each facility is able to accommodate in order to support the professional preparation component of each term.
3. To match student needs with available sites.
4. To disseminate information to the sites concerning the programme philosophy, curriculum and education guidelines.
5. To act as a resource to the sites in the planning of learning experiences and the evaluation of student performance.
6. To monitor individual student progress throughout practicum and to assist the student in developing strategies to meet his/her ongoing learning objectives throughout the programme.
7. To submit final student grades to PASC for approval.
8. To maintain a database on sites and preceptors.
9. To liaise with the Term Teams to ensure that curriculum content enhances student preparation for practicum experiences.
10. To address current issues and future directions within the profession in Ontario by sitting on the Ontario Fieldwork Coordinators of Occupational Therapy Programmes Committee (OFCOT).
11. To address current issues and future directions within the profession in Canada by sitting on the Committee of the University Fieldwork Coordinators of the Association of Canadian Occupational Therapy University Programmes (ACOTUP).
12. To address accommodation issues that affect the practicum experience.

Evaluation

Students are responsible for developing and implementing learning objectives as components of the Competency Based Fieldwork Evaluation for Occupational Therapists (CBFE-OT) (Bossers et al., 2002). The CBFE-OT serves as the basis for learning and evaluation of student performance for each placement. This helps focus the student's learning objectives, identify learning resources and establish clear evidence to demonstrate completion of the learning. Typical learning objectives may need to be interpreted somewhat differently in a role emerging versus more traditional setting. The occupational therapy profile (Canadian Association of Occupational Therapists, 2007) may be used to help focus the objective and apply appropriate activities and resources for the particular setting.

Students in REP settings are also required to complete a reflective journal related to their learning experiences. This may take on many forms and can include entries on clinical questions or challenges, reflections on critical incidents or team interactions, strategies to address learning objectives and valuable resources found or developed, etc. This journal is shared with the supervisor on a regular (at least weekly) basis and can be used as a format for remote communication and to serve to help focus the discussion with the occupational therapist at the weekly on-site supervision times. Journaling has also been a useful tool to demonstrate the student's development throughout the course of the placement. Students are also required to complete a written evaluation of the supervisor and learning setting at the conclusion of the placement. The university PPC maintains ongoing contact with all parties throughout the placement period and is available as the need arises to address learning or evaluation issues that may emerge.

Following the completion of the placement, the PCC meets with the students to obtain verbal feedback on the learning opportunity (challenges and opportunities) and to gather information that will be helpful in sustaining the educational partnership or determining whether the placement is a valuable and viable one. A similar meeting is held with the agency contacts/supervisors. A single meeting with all parties may be arranged if it is felt that open communication and honest feedback will be possible for all involved.

The model at Leeds Metropolitan University West Yorkshire, UK

At Leeds Metropolitan University, the pre-registration education of occupational therapy students is at masters level with a problem-based learning approach and has been running full cohort role emerging placements since 2006. The REP placement sits within a module which focuses on occupation, health, groups and communities. Farrow (1995) is in support of the role emerging placement being situated within the academic curriculum and advocates the establishment of a formal student project proposal that can be instigated and designed alongside university curricula activity, and then carried out on placement. Thus, the students are encouraged to think of a 'project' that they might develop whilst on placement that can demonstrate to staff and service users in the placement setting, how an occupational therapy approach or perspective might deliver positive benefits. The programme at Leeds was specifically devised to prepare the students with support from practicing occupational therapists, university academic staff and peers; most of the placements are supervised via a long arm mode of supervision from an external qualified occupational therapist, the academic staff do not usually provide the placement supervision. Students tend to be anxious about practice placements whether they are traditional or not, and preparation and planning of placements is essential for students anxieties to lessen (Spiliotopoulou, 2007).

Preparation for the role emerging practice placement

In terms of the role emerging placement at Leeds Metropolitan University, the member of staff supervising the student in the setting is referred to as the *on-site practice placement educator* (OSPPE), and the 'off-site' supervising occupational therapist is the *occupational therapy practice placement educator* (OTPPE); the roles and responsibilities are listed in Box 2.2. Once a setting is identified, an academic member of staff will visit

Box 2.2   Roles and responsibilities within the REP at Leeds Metropolitan University

The role and responsibilities of students:

- To adhere to the College of Occupational Therapists *Code of Ethics and Professional Conduct for Occupational Therapists* and the Health Professions Council *Standards of Conduct, Performance and Ethics.*
- To complete a daily time sheet.
- To use student log-book as guidance for the placement
- To liaise with both PPEs regarding any potential occupational perspective that the student foresees may be of benefit to the setting
- To be self-directed in identifying own learning needs and in seeking resources to fulfill learning outcomes
- To record reflections in the reflective diary of the role emerging placement student logbook
- To ensure that any project or role that is established is sustainable after completion of the placement
- To seek out support an guidance particularly if there is uncertainty about client/ service user risk or risk to self
- To provide informal feedback, both positive and constructive, to his/her practice placement educator/s throughout the placement.
- To evaluate and provide feedback to the university at the end of their role emerging placement.

Role and responsibilities of the on-site practice placement educator (OSPPE):

- To prepare the setting team/staff for student placement.
- To provide/oversee induction.
- To provide support and guidance to the student re-setting issues.
- To act as principle setting 'expert'.
- To liaise regularly (at least once a week) with the appropriate OTPPE. Re: student progress.
- To provide regular supervision both individually with the student and jointly with the OTPPE and student.
- To maintain communication with university staff.
- To ensure that student is not treated as 'another pair of hands' and recognise their role is as a student and not a qualified occupational therapist.
- To provide information and resources regarding relevant policies and procedures, e.g. health and safety, risk and workload management, etc.

Role and responsibilities of the occupational therapy practice placement educator (OTPPE):

- To support student to see an occupational perspective
- To support the student in identifying role of occupational therapist
- To provide professional accountability
- To provide guidance with theory into practice (clinical reasoning)
- To act as a role model for the profession
- To facilitate and support student reflection Signposts other resources for the student to learn from
- To assess the student in regards to the competencies in the CBFE
- To offer evaluation and feedback on the placement
- To ensure regular informal dialogue on performance, and one hour of 'formal' dedicated supervision per week.
- To discusses assessment outcomes and comments with the student and university staff

The role and responsibilities of university-based staff:

- To oversee and ensure the smooth running of the practice placements
- To keep the practice placement educators informed of any changes to placements

(Continued)

Box 1.2   (*Continued*)

- To provide named university educator contact details.
- To provide appropriate support for the students on practice placement, e.g. placement visit
- To ensure that the student has the opportunity to fulfil the requisite number of hours
- To provide ongoing education and support for practice placement educators.
- To oversee the monitoring and evaluation of the practice placement as an appropriate learning environment for pre-registration students.
- To ensure that the settings and learning opportunities are appropriate to achieve learning outcomes.
- To facilitate the learning from placement is enhanced within the university
- To ensure all documentation matches the requirement of the College of Occupational Therapists, World Federation of Occupational Therapists and relevant policies

---

the setting and provide written information (usually sent before the visit) proving full details about the placement objectives and philosophy. The setting staff have to accept responsibility for the student and meet health and safety requirements as well as agreeing to provide both formal and informal supervision. All the supervisors involved in the role emerging placement should attend a half-day workshop regarding the education and supervision of the student in such placements. They all have to be familiar with the assessment tool, which is standardised (Bossers et al., 2002) and is same as that for the traditional placements. The OTPPEs also meet with the OSPPEs and are encouraged to meet with the student at least formally once in the setting before the placement commences full time.

Supervision during the placement

During the placement supervision is required formally once a week, face to face between the student and both educators in the setting, as well as informally via phone or e-mail with the OTPPE. Some students use the informal supervision regularly, others are content to liaise pre-dominantly with the OSPPE and only discuss their objectives with their OTPPE when they visit each week. All supervision notes are recorded in the student's placement logbook. The students also have to complete a reflective record, which they can use to support their experiential learning and supervision.

Involving occupational therapists from the outset, both in discussing the mode of supervision for students, and also in predicting any problems, can pay dividends. Thomas et al. (2005) suggest that the 'best of both worlds' is to involve occupational therapists working in partnership with community agencies or industry, both support the student in identifying an emerging role for professional practice. The responsibility for facilitating student learning therefore is shared between the OSPPE and the OTPPE, as advocated by Fisher and Savin-Badin (2002). The model at Leeds Metropolitan University prepares the student by supporting their initial attendance at the REP setting by attending one day a week for five weeks, (to develop their project idea) and then attend full time for five weeks (see Table 2.2 timelines for placements).

Table 2.2 Timetable showing how the REP is delivered at Leeds Metropolitan University.

	Weeks	Mon	Tues	Wed	Thurs	Fri
University-based work only	1–3	Study	University-based work	University-based work	University-based work	University-based work
One-day-per-week REP embedded in the academic timetable	4–9	Study	University-based work	REP All day	University-based work + 1 hour peer group support on REP	University-based work
Five weeks fulltime	10–15	REP All day	REP All day	REP All day	REP All day	REP All day
Assessment week	16	Students finalise and hand in a formal report on the REP project that was developed with a supporting reflective evidence of learning whilst on placement				

Aims of one day a week for five weeks

- To allow the student to become gradually familiar with the setting and liaise with their peers/university staff to explore potential projects.
- To provide university-based learning to complement the placement.
- To provide opportunities to explore the experiences of placement with peers/university staff via peer group discussion groups.
- To allow the OTPPE to support the student regarding any potential ideas, and to visit the student in the role emerging setting at least once within this stage of the placement.
- To identify and develop the resources needed to assist the student when they attend full time.
- To provide opportunity for any potential problems that could impact on the service/setting and/or the student, to be identified and rectified without disruption to the placement.
- To facilitate reflective and self-directed learning, reviewed by both the PPEs and university academic staff prior to commencing full time.

Aims of five weeks full-time attendance at the REP

- To provide the student with a substantial amount of time to establish a meaningful contribution to the practice placement setting, as well as allowing opportunities for their own learning to take place.
- To include a halfway report using the placement assessment and a visit by an academic member of staff.
- To allow the student to concentrate on establishing the contribution of an occupational perspective of humans and health within the context of the needs of the setting and in constant dialogue with both PPEs.

- To offer the opportunity for the student to present a project with a view as to how it could be sustained after the student has left the placement.
- To allow the student access to resources from a variety of means including visits to other agencies, or settings to extenuate learning and experiences.

The students are prepared for the placement by a formal presentation which includes details of the REP model, their roles and responsibilities, etc; they are also given a list of the possible settings to choose from. Students are given the same information on the placement as the placement educators; they are also given some examples of previous placements and the projects that took place. They attend a peer reflective review session the day after their one-day-a-week attendance at the REP. Facilitated reflection and discussion in peer groups of the students experience on the placement once a week, helps support the student with the occupational perspective and potential project ideas. These small group discussions are led by a university academic tutor, who also supports students individually if this is required. Students can support one another and sometimes this has led to a sharing of projects, or provides collaborative working between settings.

Learning outcomes

All students have to pass a written assignment which assesses the extent to which the learning outcomes of the module were met, these learning outcomes integrate the university-based learning with the practice placement (Box 2.3), this allows the student to develop specific skills associated with innovative or less traditional occupational therapy practice. For example, the student will learn early on in the module, how to conduct a local health needs assessment, rather than a purely occupational or condition focused one.

The module assessment is a formal report of the 'project' set up within the REP setting that demonstrates the value of occupation or occupational therapy to the setting/service users. It also incorporates a reflective piece, which is drawn from the student reflective journal which they are encouraged to keep and to use to facilitate discussion and learning at formal supervision times. This project offers another advantage in that the placement setting providers have a demonstrable outcome associated with the placement. This, however, has had a mixed response in terms of the student satisfaction, with some commenting on the fact that they can become project and not placement focused (Thew et al, 2008). This is despite education and guidance given to educators that the focus of the placement is on the student's learning.

Allocation of student to placement setting

At Leeds, the students are given a choice of placement setting within the spectrum of settings offered but have to offer an explanation as to why they feel the particular setting would meet their learning needs (Table 2.3). A similar offer is made to the occupational therapy educators, as most are not connected to any of the settings. Therefore, the allocation of student to setting is based on: (i) the strength of argument from the student; (ii) whether the placement was in pairs; (iii) whether a car was required; (iv) previous

---

Box 2.3   Learning outcomes for the Leeds Metropolitan University module and REP

The student on this module will develop the following:

Knowledge
- Discuss methods of developing and facilitating therapeutic relationships.
- Identify a range of methods for assessing individuals, groups and communities
- Discuss a range of intervention approaches suitable for individuals, groups and communities.
- Recognise opportunities for the development of innovative occupational therapy services.
- Discuss occupational therapy clinical reasoning theories and models.
- Discuss the global and local factors which impact on the health of individuals, groups and communities.
- Discuss the global and local factors which impact on occupational performance.
- Discuss how and why various contexts influence occupational therapy practice.

Skills
- Develop programmes to improve/maintain an individual's capacities and abilities.
- Grade and adapt a range of occupations.
- Modify a range of environments and contexts.
- Initiate, maintain and end therapeutic relationships.
- Tailors methods and tools of intervention to ensure cultural sensitivity.
- Assess individuals, groups and communities and produce an occupation focused action plan.
- Plan and deliver occupational therapy intervention for individuals and groups.
- Outline the contribution an occupational perspective could make to current societal issues.
- Applies a range of theories and models when undertaking and reflecting on own practice.
- Utilise current evidence to develop and deliver occupational therapy.

Attitudes
- Commit to an occupational perspective of humans and health.
- Accept individual and cultural differences in occupations.
- Be confident in the contribution occupational therapy can make to issues of health and well-being.
- Value the contributions of others involved in working with clients.

---

placement experience. This latter factor is only used to avoid sending students who, for example, have already worked in paediatrics to a school setting. Students are usually, allocated into each setting in twos (as advocated by Bossers et al., 1997). This can present as a challenge to occupational therapy educators who are therefore required to not only provide long arm supervision, but to two students.

Students' evaluation of role emerging placements

Leeds Metropolitan University students appear to value the role emerging placements (Thew et al., 2008). A more recent informal evaluation below (Figure 2.1) indicates that the majority of students in 2009 felt the experience gave them confidence, helped them meet their learning outcomes and would recommend the placement to others. Where there was a negative experience (in one placement), the reasons were due to issues within

Table 2.3 Recent Leeds Metropolitan University REP settings attended by students.

Settings for REPs (Leeds)	Focus for role emerging practice
Remand prison	Working with people who have recently been placed on remand and are awaiting sentencing; many have mental health and drug-related problems
Community allotment	Working with many local groups of people who use a charity-funded allotment to grow organic food and to gain well-being
Independent living hostel	Helping those who have been living in or relying on mental health institutions for many years to develop the skills for independent community living
City library services	A service which offers people with many needs access resources to enhance literacy, confidence and self-esteem within a non-health–orientated setting
Community personality disorder service	A community-based service for people with personality disorders who are not able to access support from mainstream mental health services
Refuge detention centre	Large centre where refugees are temporarily housed awaiting decisions regarding their immigration status; these are occupationally deprived and have multiple needs
Community respiratory team	Largely nursing-based service for people living at home with severe respiratory disorders
Travellers' families education service	Services for gypsy, Roma, travellers' families who are not able to gain educative support, often occupationally deprived and alienated
Memory services – older age adults	Developing an occupation focused service for people with significant memory problems
Black health community charity	Providing mental health and well-being support particularly for those from culturally diverse and hard to reach populations in the community
Community cardiac rehabilitation service	Helping people with chronic and severe heart failure to access and participate in meaningful occupation

that setting area, and not that it was unsuitable for occupational therapy practice. Their comments echo that of previous students (Thew et al., 2008) in that:

a) they learn a great deal about the value and benefits of occupation
b) they learn more self-management skills than in a traditional placement
c) they value the autonomy and flexibility of learning
d) they are often considered 'experts' in occupation by experienced staff
e) they can find the pressure to provide a meaningful project challenging
f) they value being with a peer on placement
g) they value support from the university, and need more of it than in a traditional placement
h) there is greater scope for innovative practice
i) OSPPEs can either 'make or break' the positive experience.

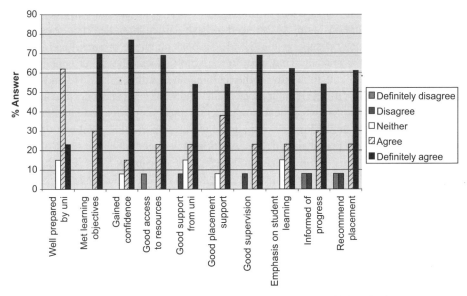

Figure 2.1   Student evaluation of their REP at Leeds Metropolitan University in 2009.

Lessons learned in establishing and facilitating REPs

Pre-registration occupational therapy student involvement in REP opportunities has resulted in many 'lessons learned' for the academic staff, the students and the supervisors. However, in the main, the experience of setting up such placements remains positively received by most who are concerned, indeed, some students particularly thrive on an REP. Overwhelmingly, the experiences in both programmes is that the non-traditional placement is a feature of both courses that is beneficial for student learning, raising awareness of contemporary issues, developing autonomy and in creating an increased awareness of what occupational therapy and/or an occupational perspective can contribute.

Ultimately, however, solid preparation of the student, on-site and off-site supervisors is essential to the success of these learning opportunities. Expectations of the placement and strategies for clear and frequent communication can eliminate confusion and misunderstandings that may result in frustration for all involved. Setting up placements in settings that often have no clear understanding of occupational therapy, requires considerable time and effort. There is a need to promote and describe occupational therapy in many of the settings. This requires a clear remit of the aims of the placement and clearly promoting the philosophy behind using the setting as a learning opportunity for the student and for the setting staff. It is important, particularly in the charity sector, to establish the role of the student as 'learner' and not a volunteer. The offer of a project that demonstrates the value of occupation or occupational therapy is useful in offering the setting something tangible in return for their support. Introductory meetings play a key role in clarifying expectations and roles, thereby reducing anxiety for all parties. Workshops can enhance that understanding and are particularly relevant in getting occupational therapists fully engaged in the long arm supervision.

Preparing appropriate supervision of the student is key to successful placements; occupational therapy supervisors may also need to have particular skills. They need to be comfortable with hands-off supervision (i.e. discussions on phone or email) and limited direct contact with the student. They need to be able to focus the direct contact time they have with the students to maximise the learning and feedback provided and obtain relevant information for the evaluation process. Off-site supervisors may need to help the student identify and implement strategies to integrate into existing teams, anticipate barriers and supports to maintaining an occupational therapy perspective, establish structure as needed and help with personal management skills, lack of confidence or sense of being overwhelmed. Providing a named contact available at the University for issues relating to clarification of roles or resolution of potential clashes of ideas is valuable to the practice setting supervisors. By establishing personal contacts via the earlier site visits, and any educational workshops and follow-up calls, are all essential in maintaining a free flow of communication and support for the student. A re-enforcement of the student learning objectives by a practice placement educator handbook has always been useful. It reminds everyone of their roles and responsibilities. The halfway visit to the student in the setting with the occupational therapy supervisor also ensures that everyone is sharing common expectations related to the placement. Many placement settings are not set up for students and may not have computers/desks, etc available, the university should make it clear that flexibility should be allowed. The students should access university resources to support the placement, and therefore their learning, as long as the students can provide evidence that they are working on behalf of the placement to develop ideas, etc. Equally, the student may have to be flexible with their hours, if the service users tend to use the setting more at weekends, the student must follow suit, taking time off like other staff. Often setting staff are keen to invite future students on placement for the following year. There is also evidence that projects that the students produce are proving influential and there have been several examples where the project of the placement has been rolled out nationally or has been implemented locally. This kind of end product has proven to the student the 'worth' of such placements. These examples can be used to promote REP to students.

Students do appear more anxious prior to the role emerging placement compared to their other more traditional placements. Students frequently move through a 'cycle' when involved in role emerging placements. Starting with *excitement* – anticipating the opportunity; *frustration* – related to what they are supposed to be doing to add the occupational therapy perspective, how do they fit into an existing team/service; *reflection on and clarification* of the potential roles for occupational therapy; _action_ – developing and implementing a plan to add to the practice environment; *satisfaction* – that they have completed their objectives. There is some evidence that a gradual slide via a one-day-a-week attendance into the full-time placement does much to lessen anxieties about going into a setting without an occupational therapist in situ (Thew et al., 2008). Just as some students thrive on such placements, some students may not benefit from REP learning experiences. Some require more structured or traditional settings and established occupational therapy roles and may be overwhelmed by the demands and more changeable nature of the REP. That said, students do appear to perform to 'type' and there is no particular change in the student's trend of placement assessment marks. Not every site necessarily has tangible benefit from the occupational therapy input. This should not be considered a failure. Students may, in fact, find this a very unique and valuable experience that can inform their future practice. Students may need assistance in identifying the transferable skills developed in these situations (e.g. completing a needs assessment, educating others about occupational therapy, reflective practice) to help them realise how this experience can be built upon in their future practice. Helping the student to make this explicit is an important step to take as part of the de-briefing discussion and group evaluation of the placement.

Agencies/programmes may not fully appreciate the contribution of occupational therapy until a few students have had placements in that setting. Conversely, many students enjoy establishing the occupational therapy role or addressing need through occupation from 'scratch' so to speak, thus allowing them the freedom from a prescribed view. Some students may need to build on each other's legacies. As the placement setting becomes more familiar with what perspectives the occupational therapist can offer, the learning opportunities and benefits may become more apparent. As a result, students may also need to be ready to educate the team in the practice setting about occupational therapy and explore ways of "marketing" the added value that the occupational therapy perspective can bring to the setting. Procuring suitable placements has become easier with each passing year. Suggestions and contacts for potential new placements arise from the students themselves, or more frequently, from existing REP settings or REP supervisors, interestingly, however, very few originate from occupational therapists working in non-mental health traditional statutory sectors.

Anecdotally, many occupational therapists, particularly in Leeds, are keen to support or supervise such placements. However, anecdotally, there have been examples of some local occupational therapists being rather sceptical and dismissive of such innovative placements. They have informally expressed their concerns to students (which have added to the student anxieties) regarding whether such a placement will be recognised by educators as being 'legitimate' occupational therapy practice hours. This can undermine the students and the reputation of REPs, however, this scepticism is not well founded, and there is increasing evidence with each year that these placements provide a rich source of education and can increase student confidence and self-directed, autonomous learning.

Conclusion and recommendations

Practice placements in the UK and Canada have been largely offered via a traditional mode. This usually involves one student being allocated per occupational therapy educator within the social and health care sector where an occupational therapist role is established. Initially, setting up REP placements are costly in terms of academic time, however, once the approach and local culture of such placements are created, subsequent procurements of placements is easier. Directly engaging and educating local practitioners, involves little more university time compared to usual/traditional placements. By disseminating the success of REPs in newsletters (such as *OT News* in the UK) and with evidence of the applicability and benefits of REP education to students in peer reviewed publications, the REP looks set to be an acknowledged permanent feature of practice education for occupational therapists. It is worrying that, despite the increasing evidence, some occupational therapists do appear to be (anecdotally) ignorant of the benefits to students and the profession of such placements. This can only be remedied by greater volumes of research and dissemination of the impact such placements can make to students' and service users' lives.

While there are differences in the models, educational and health systems in which we are working, the challenges and benefits of developing REP placements have many common features. Despite the additional administrative tasks and responsibilities inherent in this process, the value to student education and contribution to the advancement of the profession is undeniable. The true advantage to student professional development may not always be realised by the student until they are engaged in clinical practice following graduation. Benefits for all parties involved make REP experiences an ongoing focus in the education of future occupational therapy practitioners who are prepared to accept the challenge of advancing the profession.

References

Alsop, A., & Donald, M. (1996). Taking stock and taking changes: Creating new opportunities for fieldwork education. *British Journal of Occupational Therapy, 59*, 498–502.

Bossers, A., Cook, J., Polatajko, H., & Laine, C. (1997). Understanding the role emerging fieldwork placement. *Canadian Journal of Occupational Therapy, 64*, 70–81.

Bossers, A., Miller, L., Polatajko, H., & Hartley, M. (2002). *Competency Based Fieldwork Evaluation for Occupational Therapists*. Albany: Delmar.

Canadian Association of Occupational Therapists. (2007). *Profile of Occupational Therapy Practice in Canada (2007)*. Ottawa: Canadian Association of Occupational Therapists.

Casares, G.S., Bradley, K.P., Jaffe, L.E., & Lee, G.P. (2003). Impact of the changing health care environment on fieldwork education. *Journal of Allied Health, 32* (4), 246–251.

College of Occupational Therapists. (2006). *Developing the occupational therapy profession: Providing New Work-Based Learning Opportunities for Students*. College of Occupational Therapists. Guidance 4. London. COT

College of Occupational Therapists of Ontario. (1996). *Supervision of Student Occupational Therapists*. Toronto: College of Occupational Therapists of Ontario.

DeClute, J, & Ladyshewsky, R. (1993). Enhancing clinical competence using a collaborative clinical education model. *Physical Therapy, 73* (10), 683–689.

Farrow, P. (1995) Power for the profession. In: Bossers, A., Cook, J., Polatajko, H., & Laine, C. (1997). Understanding the role emerging fieldwork placement. *Canadian Journal of Occupational Therapy, 64*, 70–81.

Fieldhouse, J., & Fedden, T. (2009). Exploring the learning process on a role-emerging practice placement: A qualitative study. *The British Journal of Occupational Therapy, 72* (7), 302.

Fisher, A., & Savin-Badin, M. (2002). Modernising fieldwork, Part 2: Realising the new agenda. *British Journal of Occupational Therapy, 65*, 275–282.

Friedland, J. Polatajko, H., & Gage, M. (2001). Expanding the boundaries of occupational therapy practice through student field-work experiences: Description of a provisionally-funded community funded community development project. *Canadian Journal of Occupational Therapy, 68* (5), 301–307.

Huddleston, R. (1999). Clinical placements for the professions allied to medicine, Part 2: Placement shortages? Two models that can solve the problem. *British Journal of Occupational Therapy, 62*, 295–298.

Hook, A. Kenny, C. (2007). Evaluating role emerging placements. *OT News*, *15* (7), 25.

Jepson, J., Wells, C., & Biswas, C. (2007). The development of a distance supervision protocol for allied health profession students on practice placements in non-traditional areas. *Higher Education Academy Mini Project Report*. Available at: http://www.health. heacademy.ac.uk/projects/miniprojects/jepson.pdf. Accessed 25 March 2010.

Jung, B., Solomon, P., & Cole, B. (2005). Role-emerging placements in rehabilitation sciences. In P. Solomon, & S. Baptiste (Eds.), *Innovations in Rehabilitation Sciences Education: Educating Leaders for the Future*. Heidelberg, Germany: Springer-Verlag.

Lloyd, C., Bassett, H., & King, R. (2002). Mental health: How well are occupational therapists equipped for a changed practice environment? *Australian Occupational Therapy Journal*, *49* (3), 163–166.

Martin, J., & Daniels, R. (2007). Role emerging placements: A success Story in a climate of cutbacks. *OT News*, *15* (2), 24.

Mitchell, M.M., & Kampfe, C.M. (1990). Coping strategies used by occupational therapy students during fieldwork: An exploratory study. *The American Journal of Occupational Therapy*, *44* (6), 543–550. Cited in: Spiliotopoulou, G. (2007). Preparing occupational therapy students for practice placements: Initial evidence. *The British Journal of Occupational Therapy*, 70 (9), 384–389.

Mulholland, S., & Derdall, M. (2005). A strategy for evaluating occupational therapy students at community sites. *Occupational Therapy International*, *12* (1), 28–32.

Overton A., Clark M., & Thomas, Y. (2009). A review of non-traditional occupational therapy practice placement education: A focus on role-emerging and project placements. *British Journal of Occupational Therapy*, *72* (7), 294–301.

Prigg, A., & Mackenzie, L. (2002). Project placements for undergraduate occupational therapy students: Design, implementation and evaluation. *Occupational Therapy International*, *9* (3), 210–236.

Thew, M., Hargreaves, A., & Cronin-Davis, J. (2008). An evaluation of a role-emerging practice placement model for a full cohort of occupational therapy students. *British Journal of Occupational Therapy*. *71* (8), 348–353.

Thomas, Y., Penman, M., Williamson, P. (2005). Australian and New Zealand fieldwork: Charting territory for future practice. *Australian Occupational Therapy Journal*, *52*, 78–81.

Wilcock, J,. Sledding, F., & Kershaw, A. (2009). Role emerging placements: The educators experience. *OT News*, *17* (9), 24.

Williams, C. (2009). In at the deep end. *OT News*, *17* (9), 26.

Wood, A. (2005). Student practice contexts: Changing face, changing place. *British Journal of Occupational Therapy*, *68* (8), 375–378.

World Federation of Occupational Therapists. (2002). *Minimum Standards for Education of Occupational Therapists*. Forrestfield: World Federation of Occupational Therapists.

Part II

Current examples of emerging practice for occupational therapists

This section offers examples of how the application of occupational therapy skills and knowledge can enrich health and well-being beyond the traditional and expected modus operandi of an occupational therapist. The philosophical background to the profession of occupational therapy in the twenty-first century has never been stronger and has become more distinct from and independent of both the medical and social care models. The development of occupational science as a body of knowledge is largely responsible for this dramatic change in direction. Clearly, there will always be parallels and blurring of roles, but in the ever-competitive nature of this world, the continued confusion of what occupational therapy can offer as a profession can lead ultimately to its demise. The profession needs to demonstrate its worth and unique contribution to the health and well-being of human beings well beyond the boundaries of traditional health and social care.

The ensuing chapters demonstrate how occupational therapists have made the difference in areas that do not have any history of involvement with occupational therapy. Many of those examples indicate that occupational therapy has a significant role to play in, for example, health promotion, prevention of ill health and keeping people at work. Occupational therapists have skills in supporting people in the management of their daily lives and occupations, and in maximising quality of life. There is a strength and sense of empowerment that emerges from the fact that our profession's philosophy provides us with the knowledge and skills to follow many paths of need as indicated by those clients whom we profess to serve.

Health and social care is now embracing the idea that people should be encouraged to manage their conditions themselves, attending primary care clinics for rehabilitation or working with charities or non-statutory organisations that encourage friends, relatives and neighbours to be involved in supporting people who are unwell. Through being in 'everyday' settings, substantial health can be maintained or regained. Maintenance of treatment within institutional settings is no longer the solution of choice, and the profession needs to capitalise on these emerging trends. These chapters provide many tangible examples of innovation and initiative that serve to enhance occupational therapy involvement in non-traditional roles.

Chapter 3

Successful role emerging placements: It is all in the preparation

Yvonne Thomas & Sylvia Rodger

Introduction

Preparation of practice educators (both off-site occupational therapists and on-site non-occupational therapy staff members), placement site and students is the key to successful role emerging placements. This chapter identifies a range of strategies that will prepare students, practice educators and the placement sites and enable students to achieve learning objectives despite the absence of an on-site occupational therapy practice educator. The chapter is based on the experiences of the authors, both university staff, in facilitating such placements and evaluating role emerging placements in Queensland, Australia.

The objectives of this chapter are to:

1. Identify the preparation required to maximise placement outcomes and enhance student learning.
2. Identify the preparation and resources that students need to optimise their learning in role emerging placements (including reflection, peer support/learning and project management skills).
3. Review practice educator skills and relationships needed to support students.

In role emerging placements students need to be autonomous learners, which may be challenging for those with limited life experience and who may lack confidence. The strategies described in this chapter fall into three areas; (1) preparation and planning, (2) enabling student development, and (3) support through practice education including reflective journaling and project management skills. Supervision models and teaching and learning strategies are reviewed with regards to supporting students' learning in such placements. The chapter is informed by the results of two studies involving students', practice educators' and graduates' perceptions of role emerging placements and outlining how student performance can be enhanced during role emerging placements.

Role Emerging Occupational Therapy: Maximising Occupation-Focused Practice, 1st edition. Edited by Miranda Thew, Mary Edwards, Sue Baptiste and Matthew Molineux. © 2011 Blackwell Publishing Ltd.

Preparation is key

Ensuring that the site, practice educators and supporting staff are up to it

Regardless of setting, the success of any practice education placement requires effective communication between the student, practice educator and faculty staff (Fisher & Savin-Baden, 2002). Given the additional complexities associated with the role emerging placements, thorough, well-planned and executed preparation is particularly important. Significant preparation is required by all parties to guarantee success. The placement site must be first readied for the experience.

Prior to the placement a meeting between the university educators, the placement site and the practice educator will provide the means to clearly establish the roles and expectations of all the players. There needs to be discussion of the roles of the practice educators in relation to student supervision. These early discussions can clarify the needs and expectations of the non-occupational therapy practice educator, the occupational therapy practice educator and other staff/team members at the site, such as site managers. Discussion may include:

- how on-site staff will manage and support the day to day issues;
- responsibility of the occupational therapy practice educator for supervision of the student's performance of occupational therapy roles, tasks and responsibilities;
- the contributions from each practice educator in completing the student evaluation as required by the university.

Once the basic outline of the placement is agreed, further meetings may be needed to clarify and structure the student's role and tasks, and any expectations of student performance held by all parties. Inclusion of the student in these meeting, prior to the start of the placement, may help to orientate the student to the practice setting and to the multiple levels of supervision available. Where appropriate, a consumer representative may be included to contribute to the meeting. Including students in collaborative planning and preparation increases the value of the learning experience to students (Clarke et al., 2008).

To ensure quality learning experiences, students must be adequately prepared by providing clear expectations and guidelines, and regular communication between the student, practice educator and university educator (Overton et al., 2009). A key strategy is to schedule regular supervision times that are convenient to the student, their practice educators and the other staff at the organisation. It is important to determine the appropriate time and locations for these meetings and establish the most appropriate methods for contacting the off-site occupational therapy practice educator and the university for support. However, once these plans are established, it is important for all parties to allow room for flexibility to the schedule as required. This stresses the importance of early communication of issues as they arise and the importance of regular clarification and reassessment of expectations at various points as the placement progresses.

Practice educators, both on and off site, must be adequately prepared and it is suggested that additional education and knowledge is provided prior to undertaking supervision (Prigg & Mackenzie, 2002). For example, practice educators may be unsure of the requirements of spending time with the students when undertaking a self-directed practice education placement (Prigg & Mackenzie, 2002). Such training can assist with all aspects of practice education provision including understanding educator and student expectations and improving the student evaluation process (Prigg & Mackenzie, 2002). To this end, the Queensland Occupational Therapy Fieldwork Collaborative (QOTFC) developed a website (http://www.qotfc.edu.au) to assist practice educators in preparing for, conducting, managing and evaluating student placements. Of relevance to this chapter, the QOTFC has also developed practice tip sheets (accessible from the website) to assist practice educators with role emerging placements, some of which are summarised later in this chapter.

At the outset of the role emerging placement it is important to identify, discuss and plan possible projects and tasks for the student to undertake whilst on the placement. The projected outcomes should be flexible initially and allowed to evolve as the project progresses. Potential projects may focus on resource development, development of new initiatives/programmes, or conducting needs analyses. Including activities that involve direct client interventions may increase motivation and learning opportunities for the student. The precise needs of the practice setting can be assessed as part of the project management process, and may lead to implementation of a plan that is tailored to the individual setting. In this way, and with appropriate support, students have the potential to make a valuable contribution to organisations despite the absence of an established occupational therapy role. As the placement progresses, the students' ability to effectively implement the plan will develop through recognition of the relevant knowledge and skills they have gained during their occupational therapy training.

Preparation of the placement site should include some preliminary discussion regarding the specific areas of occupational therapy that may be relevant to the setting. This will help to provide some direction to the student and ensure the on-site staff understand the areas of the organisation that occupational therapy students will be able to contribute to. Finally, it is important to ensure that the student assessment process is appropriate to the role emerging setting and any assessment criteria that are not applicable or need to be adapted to fit the practice setting. The modification of any assessment of placement evaluation process needs attention prior to the placement commencement and student benefit from being involved in these discussions.

In summary, there are a number of key preparation considerations for role emerging placements (Overton et al., 2009):

- Establish effective communication patterns between all parties (e.g. frequency, regularity, methods).
- Brief all staff at the placement site regarding the students' role and the expectations and implications for their involvement in the placement setting.
- Conduct pre-placement interview with students, on- and off-site practice educators, and university staff member.
- Assist students to appreciate the relevance of their established skills and experiences in other settings to the role emerging placement setting.
- Use a practice education evaluation tool suitable for role emerging placements.

- Prepare the occupational therapy practice educator (located in a nearby and similar setting, nearby and different setting, or from the university) to understand his/her responsibilities and required contribution to the student's learning experience and success of the placement.

Ensuring that the student is up to it

Good preparation prior to placements has been associated with increasing student confidence and placement readiness, decreasing student anxiety and providing an enhanced learning environment (Spiliotopoulou, 2007). In the case of role emerging placements, preparations should focus on areas of anticipated professional skills development rather than focusing on clinical skills. Professional skills gained in role emerging placements include communication, organisation, project management, self-directed learning, ability to work autonomously, using initiative and obtaining professional support (Overton et al., 2009).

The nature of role emerging placements means that it is often impossible to identify specific outcomes at the beginning of the placement, and therefore students may experience a lack of direction and certainty about placement expectations from the onset. Therefore, preparation must address managing this uncertainty and applying strategies to develop placement outcomes as early as opportunities arise. To prepare students for this experience, some advice is provided in Box 3.1.

At the commencement of the placement, the students should reflect on their current level of skills and identify areas for improvement. On the basis of these reflections students should develop a learning plan in negotiation with the practice educators and the university educators. The characteristics of capable students identified by Kirke et al. (2007) are presented in Table 3.1 as a reflection tool for students and practice educators. This list of attributes applies to occupational therapy students in any model of practice education placement. Students with many of these characteristics will do well wherever they are placed, however, it is important to note that students rarely demonstrate all of these qualities. As a reflection tool the intention is to raise both students' and practice educators' awareness of the skills already possessed and those that require further development and refinement during the placement.

Great expectations – understanding hopes and concerns for an unfamiliar model of placement

It is realistic to expect that both students and practice educators may have desired outcomes as well as concerns before embarking upon the role emerging placement. It is important to recognise and validate these feelings, and for the students and their practice educators to collaboratively plan the placement so that desired goals are achieved and potential issues are pre-empted.

In a recent study of students and practice educators undertaking role emerging placements in Queensland (Rodger et al., 2009), it was found that prior to the placement

Box 3.1: General Guidelines for Students

1. Consider a role emerging placement as an opportunity to challenge yourself and to create an occupational therapy role within a workplace. Students have previously reported feeling they were doing something important by establishing a new role within an organisation and were able to develop an occupational therapy role with their own unique 'slant'.
2. Be prepared to work independently. You will be in the unique position of being able to work autonomously and be creative in your interpretation of the occupational therapy role.
3. Use your supervision time wisely. Prepare for supervision sessions, ask questions, be organised and be prepared to relate what you have been seeing at the workplace to your occupational therapy models
4. Be prepared to relate everything you see and do to your occupational therapy models/frameworks/ principles to get the best experience from this type of placement. Nobody else is going to do this for you and this will ensure you are being proactive in your learning.
5. Consider the role emerging placement as a unique opportunity to really develop team working skills and your understanding of a diverse range of perspective of other team members.
6. Enjoy yourself!!!! Students have previously described these placements as 'challenging' and 'exciting'. Enjoy the contact you have with clients in this experience – which will help you to understand them as people (Bossers et al., 1997).
7. Be proud to be an occupational therapist. This placement provides you with an opportunity to expand the role and increase the profile of occupational therapy, and will help you to develop your professional identity.

(adapted from http://www.qotfc.edu.au, Clinical Education Resource Kit for Mental Health Placements p. 20) accessed 4 March 2009.

commencement students were generally optimistic and believed that their impending placement would be advantageous for developing professional skills and confidence and interest in a new area of practice. Students and practice educators similarly predicted that the role emerging placement would offer a 'broader experience', with increased autonomy and independence identified as the key benefits. However, both students and practice educators harboured concerns. Students' main concerns included potential disadvantage from having no on-site occupational therapist practice educator, contending with conflicting or contradictory views from multiple practice educators, difficulty in educating site staff about the occupational therapy role and limited opportunities to develop clinical, discipline-specific knowledge. The absence of an on-site occupational therapist was also highlighted by practice educators as a major concern. It appeared that prior to the placement starting, all players held similar expectations of the roles of student, practice educator and university, outlined in Table 3.2.

This study also demonstrated that by the end of their role emerging placement, students clearly understood the potential for role emerging placements to raise the profile of occupational therapy services in organisations/institutions without a previously established occupational therapy role. Students' responses indicated that they appreciated the opportunity to act as pioneers and further develop occupational therapy services. Students reported that the placement had enabled development of skills including initiative,

Table 3.1 Self-reflection checklist for students (adapted from Kirke et al., 2007).

Desired attributes	Reflection questions for students
Self-directed learner	How do I learn? Do I rely on others? Can I direct my own learning? How can I take more responsibility?
Knowledge seeker	Do I naturally seek knowledge or wait to be told? How might I become more self-directed with this?
Applies theory to practice	What do I need to do to apply theory to practice? What theory do I need to know?
Seeks out feedback	How do I find out how I am going? What questions might I ask to obtain feedback? When is the best time to do this?
Demonstrates initiative	How can I demonstrate what I have done of my own accord? How do I know that what I have done is OK? What am I allowed/not allowed to do independently in this setting? Are there any risk/safety issues?
Flexible with learning	How can I be more flexible with what I learn? How can I adapt/transfer learning from other placements?
Adapts to the agency environment	What do I need to do to 'fit in' within this environment? What is important in terms of the social dynamics, work ethic, team functioning in this workplace?
Displays insight into strengths and weaknesses	What do I consider my strengths and challenges coming into this placement? What are my learning goals? How might I meet these?
Presents professionally	How might I demonstrate professionalism in this environment? What are the requirements?
Well organised	Am I naturally organised? If not how can improve this? If so, what do I do to stay on track and be organised? What works for me?
Enthusiastic	In terms of my personality, how do I demonstrate my interest and enthusiasm for what I am doing?
Interacts well with staff and clients	What opportunities do I have for interaction? What do I need to consider when interacting with staff? How is this different to client interaction?
Recognises own and educator's needs	What reflection do I need to do on situations that indicate my learning needs and any needs of my educator? For example, is he/she pressured for time, having a pressured day, is not well, had a crisis on the way to work?
Enjoys challenge	Am I someone who seeks out challenge? Or do I like to play it safe? How do I manage when out of my comfort zone?
Acknowledges limitations and mistakes	What is my natural reaction when I make a mistake? How might I handle this in this work context?
Constructs meaning out of opportunities	How do I make the most of opportunities? What do I need to do to help make sense of experiences?
In summary	What do I consider my learning strengths? What do I consider as areas for development during the placement?

Table 3.2 Expectations for student, practice educator and university roles prior to role emerging placements (Rodger et al., 2009).

Student role	Practice educator role	University role
Demonstrate initiative in the workplace	Support the student	Support both student and practice educator
Be prepared to learn	Provide learning opportunities in a safe environment	Be readily available and easily accessible
Be willing to seek and respond to feedback	Advocate for the student Facilitate interaction and collaboration	

time management and self-management. Significantly, the students realised that the skills learned whilst undertaking their role emerging placement were applicable to other areas of occupational therapy (Rodger et al., 2009).

Another recent study of interest (Clarke et al., 2008) explored graduates' experiences of role emerging placements and their perceptions of the experiences gained in role emerging placements after being in the workforce for one year. Graduates in this study recognised the importance of the professional skills in comparison to clinical skills. Similar to the students in the study by Rodger et al. (2009), these graduates reflected that the role emerging placement experience offered a valuable opportunity to develop the occupational therapy role and prepared them for working in a variety of less familiar settings including remote areas, socially disadvantaged communities, mental health, refugee health and research. Despite noting the challenge of learning without direct access to an occupational therapist whilst on placement, the graduates endorsed the use of role emerging placements in combination with other more conventional placements. Some of the benefits and limitations of role emerging placements identified in the literature are summarised in Table 3.3.

Enabling student development whilst undertaking a role emerging placement

A number of learning strategies to optimise student learning experiences whilst on a role emerging placement, are discussed in this section.

Table 3.3 Benefits and limitations of role emerging placements (2009).

Benefits	Limitations
Client is perceived as a person Clinical reasoning and self-reflection are well developed	Less development of clinical skills Supervision Issues
Professional/personal development (may include cultural competence)	Knowledge of professional role at the outset
Potentialrole development	Student Evaluation may not cover such placements adequately

Students need to appreciate contextual differences

When a placement is hosted by an organisation or community unfamiliar with occupational therapy services, understanding the context of the role emerging placement becomes critical to student success. The context of health and social services are addressed within education curricular along with common theoretical models and organisational frameworks. However, role emerging placements frequently occur in organisations that promote socio-political change and are based on alternative models and frameworks. Therefore, in order to gauge and explore the potential contribution of occupational therapy in these settings, occupational therapy students need to be prepared to observe, understand and interpret the goals of the organisations through a professional occupational lens. This forms much of their early learning experiences within the role emerging placement. The challenge for students then is to marry their understanding of the organisational framework to their occupational perspective in order to create occupational opportunities for service users.

To date, the locations for role emerging placements in Queensland have included retail pharmacies, youth justice and detention services, local town council offices, in patient wards, clubhouses, community support groups, nursing homes, indigenous health services and refugee organisations. In each case the organisations have undertaken the placement without allocation of specific funding to support the student activities and been generally unaware of the breadth and potential of occupational therapy services.

Students need a plan to enable personal learning

Whilst careful and thorough preparation of all players in the placement is key to successful student learning experiences, it is unrealistic to expect students to embark upon an unfamiliar model of placement without some sense of trepidation. Galvaan's (2006) discussion of the experience of supervising students on role emerging placements in mainstream South African schools suggests that no amount of preparation can prevent students from possibly feeling a disjuncture or sense of fragmentation, ". . . characterised by frustration and anger and the need for the right answers" (Savin-Baden, 2000, cited by Galvaan, 2006, p. 108). Fragmentation occurs when the student's values and beliefs are challenged or threatened by the unfamiliar culture of the placement setting, and consequently brings a sense of uncertainty. It is expected that the role emerging placement experience will lead students to question: *'what has occupational therapy (or what have I) got to offer here?'* If students are unable to align the focus of their placement with their future practice, then their professional identity and values may be compromised. Therefore, it is vital that when such experiences occur during the role emerging placement students explore these through a reflective process.

Together, practice educators and students embark upon a learning goal to facilitate the student's transition in knowledge from 'not knowing' to 'knowing how' to 'knowledge application' (Galvaan, 2006). Some students may not find this journey of discovery enjoyable, particularly if they are unsettled by the feeling of uncertainty. The practice educator needs to guide the students in identifying and discovering what they need to know regarding their own beliefs and values, which will subsequently enhance insight into their ability to work effectively within the situation. From our own observations, it appears that students will benefit from taking time to revisit and reconsider some of the foundational ideas of occupational therapy, to facilitate their progress forward from the experience of disjuncture. Rather than pressuring students to immediately develop a detailed plan for learning, it is recommended that the students take time to explore their frustrations, to review their assumptions about occupational therapy, and how they can meet the needs of the individuals they are working with. Students engaged in role emerging placements are encouraged and supported to use reflection to explore and potentially reframe their personal stance (i.e. the way students view themselves and their profession) in the face of a confronting and unfamiliar situation.

Students need to develop project management skills

An element of the role emerging placement that is quite a departure from more conventional placement models is the students' exposure to and participation in collaboration between the university and their host organisation and their involvement in reporting the placement outcomes of their project upon conclusion of the placement. Hence rather than fulfilling the typical roles of occupational therapy apprentice or learner, the student also performs the role of project manager. The five key processes and activities of project management as they relate to role emerging placements (Rosenau, 1998; Project Management Institution, 2000) are presented in Table 3.4.

Students need to engage in a continuous process of reflection

Reflective learning is transformative, leads to new understandings and is an essential component of professional practice in occupational therapy (Brown & Ryan, 2003). Reflection has been reported to assist in the development of clinical skills (Ciaravino, 2006) and increase the students' awareness of strengths and challenges, especially in relation to interactions with other people. In role emerging placements, reflection is considered particularly important as it encourages students to recognise their own achievements and progress their learning by exploring events that occur in the absence of an occupational therapy practice educator. Students' reflections are likely to highlight the differences in learning outcomes of role emerging versus conventional placements in clinical settings. Conventional placements within a clinical environment emphasise scientific reasoning. On the contrary, within the role emerging placement, procedural knowledge (knowing what to do) is complemented by subjective knowledge (knowing if you can do it) to determine whether practice is competent and ethical (Higgs et al., 2004). The students' ability to deal with the complexity of the placement requires that they gather essential information via narrative (the clients'/staff members' story) and pragmatic (the practical considerations) reasoning skills. The resource guide for role emerging placements developed by Bossers et al. (1997) recommends that students should reflect on the following aspects of skill development (Box 3.2).

Early attempts by students to reflect on their learning and skill development should be actively encouraged by the educator with positive feedback and genuine enquiry. Until there is a sense of partnership and trust within the relationship, practice educators

Table 3.4 Project management in role emerging placements: guide for students (adapted from Dwyer et al., 2004).

Stages of project management	Application to role emerging placements
Initiating (definition)	Although the placement has been initiated through the university and the agency, once you accept the placement you will need to discover as much as possible about the project and the expectations of all stakeholders. The initiating phase will include a needs analysis and will depend on your understanding the way that the agency currently works. During this first phase, make times to talk to as many people as possible about the organisation and the current needs in order to define the project. Do not expect to be able to define the project in the first few days.
Planning (planning)	Remember the needs analysis is the start, and so the second stage is in developing a plan,tentatively at the start, that will help you to progress with the project. Setting some initial goals will help you to focus your efforts; however, it will be essential to share your thoughts and to get feedback on the goals as you develop them. The initial plan may include identifying resources or observing processes that will help you to further clarify the project goals and outcomes. The specific goals of the project may not be identified until you have clarified what is possible and what is not realistic in the setting.
Executing (leading)	Once you have clarified the goals and potential outcomes of the project, you need to take a proactive role in ensuring its success. This will mean collaboration with others and motivating others to work with you on the project. It may include recruiting clients or other staff. If you are working with a fellow student you may be able to divide the key tasks between you or to develop a joint approach to leading the project. Leading requires that you remain positive in your approach, appear confident in your abilities to manage the project and encourage others to contribute to its success.
Controlling (monitoring)	Now you are actively involved in the project you need to take time to ensure that progress is being made and that goals will be achieved on time. At this point you may discover that the goals need to be adjusted because of unforeseen barriers or that additional goals need to be added in order to achieve the most effective outcomes. Once people can see that you are achieving outcomes they may ask you to do more. You will need to carefully balance the opportunities to do more with the need to complete the original task. Using checklists and updating documentation will help you to monitor progress.
Closing (completing)	Before you can leave the setting you must make sure that everything has been completed and that you have communicated the outcomes to everyone concerned. Plan the last week effectively to ensure that there is time for feedback to be given and that final adjustments can be made to the project in response to the feedback given. Do not leave everything to the end, prepare for finishing well in advance and make sure everyone knows that your time and your project is coming to an end. Before you leave, let people know about the benefits and challenges of the experience from your perspective.

Box 3.2 Facilitating Student Reflectivity (adapted from Bossers et al., 1997, pp.19–22)

- Role Identity
  - including reflection on the general role of the student at the beginning and at the end of the placement
  - the perception of agency staff of the role of occupational therapy
  - the role of occupational therapy at the end of the placement
- Role Development
  - identification of theories relevant to setting
  - method for setting goals
  - factors that hinder and help progress
  - skills required to overcome challenges
  - legislation and service models that guide practice
  - formulating recommendations for the future
- Clinical Reasoning Skills (in relation to client contact)
  - evidence-based practice (what is known?)
  - tacit knowledge (what is sensed?)
  - procedural knowledge(what is done?)
  - knowledge gaps (what is not yet known?)
- Critical Enquiry
  - assessment of current practice and literature
  - reflecting on and being accountable for decisions
  - critically appraising own work and soliciting input from others
- Communication Skill (with clients, agency staff and peers)
  - use of professional language
  - establishing rapport
  - assertive communication
  - listening skills and getting feedback
  - written skills
- Professionalism
  - personal strengths
  - coping strategies
  - creativity/flexibility
  - team building
  - ethical issues
  - ability to take responsibility

---

should suspend judgement and direct critique as this may discourage the students from risking further disclosure. When students identify challenges they are experiencing in the placement, practice educators need to respond positively by framing the problem as a necessary learning step in their passage to becoming a better professional. Many situations that students encounter in role emerging placements are similar to graduate experiences and consequently will provide valuable preparation for future practice. Should the student become frustrated by the process, encouraging reflection on the cause of emotions is likely to be more effective than attempting to alleviate the frustration by offering quick and simple solutions.

Supporting the practice educator whilst undertaking a role emerging placement

Practice educators need to recognise the fears, doubts and misconceptions of students

Lack of confidence is a predominant characteristic of occupational therapy students at all stages of training and in graduating occupational therapists, although insecurities differ between first and final year students (MacKenzie, 2002). The value of establishing relationships based on clear communication between the student and practice educator cannot be underestimated. Practice educators will need to assist students to overcome their initial self-doubt and recognise and utilise their abilities during the placement. Providing opportunities for briefing and debriefing has been reported to expose and ameliorate students' self-doubt and concern, whilst additionally providing opportunities to engage in reflection that will evaluate and validate their learning progress (MacKenzie, 2002).

Some students will attempt to alleviate their anxiety by determining an immediate course of action that will keep them busy but may not be appropriate to the setting. Students may justify their 'grand plans' in terms of traditional roles observed in other settings which have yet to be tested in the novel context of the role emerging placement. If such a situation arises, the practice educator may need to encourage the students to first clearly communicate their ideas with the organisation's staff and clients and seek feedback before committing to a decision. Practice educators may find it more challenging to deal with 'overly confident' students than students lacking confidence. Both situations demand high levels of empathy and understanding and the ability to mentor the student through the period of uncertainty and discomfort.

Practice educators need to possess specific supervision skills and establish a learning partnership

A Canadian study of the impact of a university employed practice educator on the experience of independent community placements (Mulholland & Derdall, 2005) found that students and the community sites most valued the following practice educator activities:

- provision of support,
- provision of information,
- liaison between the site and the university and
- identification of the occupational therapy perspective and role.

Feedback from students in this study demonstrated that the most valued qualities of their practice educator was ability to assist the students to identify, understand and develop their role at the community site, and guiding the students to set learning objectives and learn skills relevant to occupational therapy practice. Students appreciated the ongoing support from their practice educators and discussion of strategies to improve their performance, such as practical advice to deal with difficult situations, discussing ideas in greater detail and identifying resources that may be of assistance to the students (Mulholland & Derdall, 2005). Whilst these roles and qualities would also be of value in other placements, there is less time for direct contact with students within the role emerging placement. Hence how the practice educator addresses these aspects is significant.

Practice educators in role emerging placements must therefore tread a careful line between encouraging students to develop autonomy and independence and providing direct supervision (Bartholomai & Fitzgerald, 2007). It is necessary for the practice educators to engage the students in careful discussion about their preliminary ideas and plans and provide the students with an opportunity to review and reassess the situation in light of feedback. Students should be assisted to find the answers to their questions about the role of occupational therapy and their capacity to meet the demands of this role. If the practice educator assists the students in making explicit links between the challenges and opportunities of the placement in relation to occupational theory and frameworks, this will enhance the students' understanding of their role and increase their confidence to fulfil the perceived needs of the organisation. Practice educators from one study (Rodger et al., 2009) were pleased to report the growth in the occupational therapy role developed by the students and to witness the students' introduction of programmes beneficial to clients that would have otherwise not occurred. While the practice educators were concerned about the lack of physical proximity to their students, they gratefully acknowledged the contribution and support of other agency staff and support provided by the universities in assuming their new roles. In this study, time commitments required for the role emerging placements were met with mixed reactions (Rodger et al., 2009). Reports indicated that different amounts of time were invested for on-site compared to off-site practice educators, that off-site educators were required to increase the content in their tutorials and that additional time was allocated for reflection. Off-site occupational therapists reported that since their time with students was limited they felt that their sessions were critical and required significant planning. Conversely, there was an expectation that students would also devote time to preparing/planning for these supervision sessions. Practice educators felt that since this role was a departure from traditional placement supervision it required them to develop new skills.

Practice educators need to be prepared to handle more than one student

Frequently two or more students are assigned to a role emerging placement. Our experience indicates that role emerging placements generally work best when there are at least two students on placement together (Rodger et al., 2009). When students are provided the opportunity to work together, they can increase each other's confidence, share ideas, strategise together and engage in self-directed learning (Martin et al., 2004). Given the lack of an on-site occupational therapist, students can collaborate to: (1) troubleshoot ideas, (2) brainstorm, debrief and discuss what they are doing using occupational therapy terminology, and (3) provide peer support and supervision. The practice educator may elect to use collaborative supervision sessions and strategies to enhance learning. This approach includes peer learning and peer support (Martin et al., 2004). Accordingly, group supervision strategies in collaborative practice education should aim to facilitate peer learning and enhance clinical reasoning (Bartholomai & Fitzgerald, 2007). Practice educators can encourage collaborative learning by teaching students 'peer coaching' strategies (Ladyskewsky, 2006). Two factors are key for this process: constructing the learning experience so that it requires positive interdependence (i.e. the need to work together in order to meet joint goals) and individual accountability (i.e. defining the tasks that each student must achieve). Also considered beneficial for students' development of collaboration skills are exposing them to small group skills and encouraging reflection on the group process. Further advice regarding developing students' skills in peer assisted learning can be found at http://www.qotfc.edu.au.

Students also identified a number of factors which they believed were beneficial to their learning whilst on role emerging placements, including (Rodger et al., 2009):

- Company of at least one other student to provide a source of specific and general support.
- An off-site occupational therapist who acts as a role model.
- Trialling new activities/plans such as running groups without 'someone over their shoulder'.
- Being prepared for and making the most of formal supervision sessions.
- Support from staff at the placement site (e.g. nurse unit manager).
- Cooperation from the other team members at the placement site.
- Practice educators who were supportive of students' learning styles.

Conclusion

The role emerging placement can be an exciting and challenging learning experience for both students and their practice educators. This chapter has outlined some of these benefits and challenges, and further highlighted the careful preparation required for students, practice educators, the university and the placement site in order for these placements to successfully meet students' learning outcomes. We have emphasised that the role of practice educators and the university is to facilitate students' development of professional skills including project management skills, reflection skills and effective utilisation of peer support. Educators must aid students in transferring the professional and generic skills acquired through the curriculum and earlier placements to the role emerging setting. In addition, we have identified a useful self-reflection checklist for students, applied project management skills to the role emerging placement setting and provided useful links to web-based resources for students, universities and practice educators.

References

Bartholomai, S., & Fitzgerald, C. (2007). The collaborative model of fieldwork education: Implementation of the model in a regional hospital rehabilitation setting. *Australian Occupational Therapy Journal, 54*, S23–S30.

Bossers, A., Polatajko, H., Conor-Schisler, A., & Gage, M. (1997). *A Resource Guide for Role Emerging Community Placements in Occupational Therapy*. London, Canada: School of Occupational Therapy, Faculty of Health Sciences, The University of Western Ontario.

Brown, G., & Ryan, S. (2003). Enhancing reflective abilities interweaving reflection into practice. In G. Brown, S. Esdaile & S. Ryan (Eds.), *Becoming an Advanced Health Care Practitioners* (pp. 118–144). Edinburgh, UK: Butterworth.

Ciaravino, E. A. (2006). Student reflections as evidence of interactive clinical reasoning skills. *Occupational Therapy in Health Care, 20* (2), 75–88.

Clarke, M., Overton, A., & Thomas, Y. (2008). An evaluation of non-traditional occupational therapy fieldwork experiences: Role emerging (project) placements. Occupational Therapists Board of Queensland (unpublished report).

Dwyer, J., Stanton, P., & Theissen, V. (2004). Why project management? In J. Dwyer, P. Stanton, & V. Theissen (Eds.), *Project Management in Health and Community Settings* (pp. 3–22). Crows Nest, NSW: Allen and Unwin.

Fisher, A., & Savin-Baden, M. (2002). Modernising fieldwork, Part 2: Realising the new agenda. *British Journal of Occupational Therapy, 65*, 275–282.

Galvaan, R. (2006). Role emerging settings, service learning and social change. In T. Lorenzo, M. Duncan, H. Buchanan, & A. Alsop (Eds.), *Practice and Service Learning in Occupational Therapy: Enhancing Potential in Context* (pp. 103–117). Chichester, UK: Whurr.

Higgs, J., Andersen, L., & Fish, D. (2004) Practice knowledge – its nature, sources and contexts. In J. Higgs, B. Richardson, & M. A. Dahlgren (Eds.), *Developing Practice Knowledge for Health Professionals*. Edinburgh: Butterworth-Heinemann.

Kirke, P., Layton, N., & Sim, J. (2007). Informing fieldwork design: Key elements to quality in fieldwork education for undergraduate occupational therapy students. *Australian Occupational Therapy Journal, 54*, S13–S22.

Ladyskewshy, R. (2006). Building cooperation in peer coaching relationships: Understanding the relationship between reward structure, learner preparedness, coaching skill and learning engagement. *Physiotherapy, 92* (1), 4–10.

MacKenzie, L. (2002). Briefing and debriefing of student fieldwork experiences: Exploring concerns and reflecting on practice. *Australian Occupational Therapy Journal, 49* (2), 82–92.

Martin, M., Morris, J., Moore A. P., Sadlo, G., & Crouch, V. (2004) Evaluating practice education models in occupational therapy: Comparing 1:1 2:1 and 3:1 placements. *British Journal of Occupational Therapy, 67* (5), 192–200.

MulholLand, S., & Derdall, M. (2005). A strategy for supervising occupational therapy students at community sites. *Occupational Therapy International, 12* (1), 28–43.

Overton, A., Clarke, M. & Thomas, Y. (2009) A review of non-traditional occupational therapy practice placement education: a focus on role-emerging and project placements. *British Journal of Occupational Therapy, 72* (7), 294–301.

Prigg, A., & Mackenzie, L. (2002). Project placements for undergraduate occupational therapy students: Design, implementation and evaluation. *Occupational Therapy International, 9* (3), 210–236.

Project Management Institution. (2000). *A Guide to the Project Management Body of Knowledge.* Pennsylvania: PMI.

Rodger, S., Thomas, Y., Holley, S., Springfield, E., Broadbridge, J., Greber, C., McBryde, C., Hawkins, R., & Banks, R. (2009). Increasing the occupational therapy mental health workforce through innovative practice education: Evaluation of an innovative practice education placement trial in mental health. *Australian Occupational Therapy Journal.*

Rosenau, M. D. J. (1998). *Project Management for Health Care Professionals.* New York: Butterworth.

Spiliotopoulou, G. (2007). Preparing occupational therapy students for practice placements: Initial evidence. *British Journal of Occupational Therapy, 70* (9), 384–388.

Chapter 4

The student experience of a role emerging placement

Philippa Gregory, Lydia Quelch & Elisha Watanabe

Introduction

This chapter describes role emerging practice from the personal perspective of students in both the United Kingdom (UK) and Canada. Their experiences, thoughts and feelings, outcomes of learning and how the role emerging practice experience has shaped their subsequent professional practice are shared. As a student occupational therapist, professional practicum opportunities are a cornerstone of comprehensive clinical education. Academic coursework provides the foundation and essential scaffolding on which a substantial portion of our professional knowledge and expertise is built; this is where the theories and principles that underpin the profession are tied to real-world practice. While the merits of didactic education cannot be disputed, no number of classroom hours can replace the invaluable learning that is derived from hands-on, experiential opportunities in the context of contemporary clinical practice. The benefits of practicum education are self-evident. As students, practice placements represent our proverbial 'bread and butter', the ability to engage, interact, and do. It is through clinical practice placements that our professional identities and values are largely moulded and shaped, a reference point and lens from which we will inevitably draw as we enter into our own practice and negotiate the first several years as new clinicians.

As a consequence of national health reform, shifting demographics and a constantly changing socio-political climate, the breadth of placement options available to students has expanded to capture both the diversity and versatility of the profession (Thew et al., 2008). Hospital- and facility-based care remains a mainstay of the profession and carries with it a clearly delineated, well-established role. However, as the health care system strives to respond and adapt to ever-changing needs, a growing number of opportunities for service delivery in the community and with underserved populations has emerged to complement the more traditional, 'role-established' placements (Bossers et al., 1997, p. 71). With the sustainability of any profession demanding flexibility, creativity and a willingness to explore novel, perhaps unconventional ground, role emerging practice placements are proving to be an avenue for both rewarding student education and the expansion of occupational therapy practice (Thew et al., 2008).

Role Emerging Occupational Therapy: Maximising Occupation-Focused Practice, 1st edition. Edited by Miranda Thew, Mary Edwards, Sue Baptiste and Matthew Molineux. © 2011 Blackwell Publishing Ltd.

Experience from the United Kingdom

Two students from the UK experienced consecutive placements at a Travellers Education Service in the North of England. The aim of the Travellers Education Service is to provide links with Traveller communities, supporting individuals in those communities and promoting equal rights. This is achieved through a combination of encouraging access to education, promoting educational achievement and working closely with agencies to enhance and diversify their provision for Travellers. Carrying out consecutive placements, both students were actively involved in the development and implementation of a project titled 'Futures'. The purpose of this project was to promote self-development and self-esteem in young adults from Travelling communities. The ultimate goal was to devise and administer a course that would provide young adults, not in employment, education or training, with the support and direction they required regarding their futures.

Gypsy Travellers, also identified more specifically as Gypsies, Travellers, Romanies or Romas, were officially recognised as an ethnic minority in the UK only in 1976 (Race Relations Act, 1976). This, in itself, emphasises the limited understanding and acknowledgment of what is essentially a culturally unique ethnic group. Due to their chosen nomadic lifestyle, Travellers can be marginalised and isolated from services that are readily available to many other communities or individuals (Bancroft et al., 1996). This can lead to segregation and further division from society. This isolation can come as a result of prejudice and/or as a result of a lack of understanding of the needs and desires of Travellers. Like other individuals, Travellers require access to health care, housing, utilities, education, work and leisure occupations. Without this access, Travellers may be placed at a disadvantage in the wider community and this can have a negative impact on their health and well-being. Within the Travellers' culture individual lifestyles can understandably vary. Experiences from this placement exposed both students to Travellers living in static caravans on council approved sites, Travellers living in council-owned and rented houses within the city and roadside Travellers leading a particularly nomadic way of life. A consistent perspective from many of the service users was a view that traditional approaches to education did not match their own cultural needs. Both occupational therapy students observed that Traveller youth attendance at school was generally erratic and a lack of formal education ultimately placed individuals at a disadvantage with regards to future employment and accessing necessary services within wider society.

A number of practitioners, working in the field of occupational science and occupational therapy, have identified risk factors that impede occupational engagement and subsequently impact on health and well-being. Wilcock (1998) introduced the term, occupational deprivation, referring to the deprivation of occupational choice and subsequent sense of exclusion. Occupational deprivation can be caused by a number of external factors including social, political, cultural, economic or environmental influences. Travellers can experience feelings of isolation and negativity as a consequence of the lack of understanding or appreciation of their way of life from the wider community. A further risk factor impacting on young Travellers in particular is the notion of occupational imbalance. Wilcock (1998) explained this as a lack of balance of occupations within which an individual engages, potentially leading to experiences of ill health. It has been observed that many young Travellers have negative experiences of school due to cultural, social and institutional issues (Every Traveller Child Matters, 2007). It may be the case that they do not feel included, school is not meaningful for them, or it is inaccessible due to issues surrounding language or literacy. As a result, these young Travellers can develop limited daily structure and this can promote inactivity. Potentially this can reduce opportunities to try new experiences and ultimately lead to low self-esteem due to limited occupational engagement. People need challenging and meaningful productive roles to develop a sense of competence and self-esteem (Minato & Zemke, 2004).

The occupational issues faced by young Travellers provide a good overall example of occupational injustice. Wilcock and Townsend (2000) explained occupational injustice as an inequity with regards to the occupations available to individuals and communities. Due to the nature of Travellers' lifestyles and ethnicity, society is not always sympathetic to their occupational choices and needs. Through a variety of means the Travellers Education Service attempts to address some of these issues through adapted forms of education and advocacy of Travellers rights. The Travellers Education Service did not specifically address occupational risk factors. However, during the role emerging placements the students were able to identify and apply these concepts using evidence-based practice.

Philippa's account

As the first occupational therapy student to work within this setting, I was initially faced with the challenges of identifying and communicating the role of an occupational therapist. I was, however, encouraged by people's genuine interest in occupational therapy and what it had to offer their service. The employees were highly supportive and welcoming, providing numerous opportunities to observe their practice. This made my induction into the placement an enjoyable and stimulating experience and helped me explore and identify occupational possibilities within the setting. It was helpful that, as part of my course, I was required to complete a project exploring an occupational perspective of humans and health in this particular service. I was also required to produce something tangible, which could be left to support the work I had completed on the placement. This provided me with direction and a framework for practice. Additionally, the organisation of the course module supported my experience as the initial stage of the placement involved only one day a week, for a period of five weeks, working in the placement setting, before the full-time, five-week placement began. The rest of the working week in the initial five-week period was spent at university reflecting with my peers and consolidating my learning. These university sessions provided me with the opportunity to explore project ideas and share positive and negative experiences in a supported environment, thus promoting my confidence in the work I was undertaking.

In the early stages of my placement I had recognised the limited support available for young Travellers. My observation was supported by research highlighting that this is an isolated group (Derrington & Kendall, 2004). The Travellers Education Service had been offered funding to develop opportunities for this group and I identified the potentially valuable input an occupational therapy student could provide. My personal involvement in 'Futures' was therefore working in conjunction with staff from the Travellers

Education Service in the preliminary stages of the project. This included research, course development and promotion within the Travelling community. Furthermore, to address the requirements of my course module, it was my aim to develop a resource file and leaflet so that staff and service users could be signposted to and readily access other facilities offering support in the community. The biggest challenge I faced was achieving access to appropriate service users. Travellers can encounter marginalisation (Lomax et al., 2000; Goward et al, 2006) and therefore understandably show sensitivity to intervention from individuals outside their community. However, through working closely with staff from the service and utilising opportunities to develop rapport with Traveller families I was given the chance to engage with young Travellers and could therefore explore specific occupational needs. Some examples of how this was achieved were through shadowing staff from the service as they visited temporary Travellers' sites and networking with Travellers already working for the service. Once the links were created I could meet young Travellers in their own homes and afford them the opportunity to openly explore ongoing needs and issues in a safe environment. This provided me with the necessary information to develop an approach to address these needs. In addition to interviewing young Travellers, I worked alongside other professionals in a steering group forum where I clarified research findings and offered ideas regarding development of the 'Futures' course. I also networked with local services and established links with individuals interested in supporting the 'Futures' project. It was evident that sustaining change was not something that could be realistically achieved on a short practice placement of only six weeks. However, the fact that I was able to elucidate and justify my project goals meant I was supported by all individuals involved. They understood that my research and promotion was the foundation for the wider project and if this were to continue successfully it would be necessary for further work to be completed. They appreciated that if I finalised all aspects of my work and handed over my research effectively, the 'Futures' project could continue and the intended course for young Travellers could go ahead. Furthermore, I was confident that I had encouraged understanding of the occupational aspects of the project, so could be certain an occupational focus would remain following the completion of my placement.

Having an on-site practice placement educator within the service and a long-arm (off-site) occupational therapy educator providing weekly supervision meant I was continually offered invaluable support. It has been suggested that 'long-arm supervision' in occupational therapy practice placements encourages the development of skills and promotes clear understanding of the role of occupational therapy (Daniels, 2007). This approach to supervision and practice placement education certainly allowed me to develop my professional skills independently and encouraged me to remain focused on the occupational elements of the project.

On reflection, I feel my role emerging placement provided me with a significant sense of autonomy. Working in an environment with no specific role-profile meant I had a professional responsibility to ensure the work I carried out reflected the valuable input an occupational therapist can offer. Furthermore, to accurately promote the role, I had to show increased confidence in my ability and present a sound working knowledge of the theory that underpins practice. The role emerging placement itself also offered me an invaluable opportunity to work in a unique setting with an interesting and culturally diverse client group.

Lydia's experience

As the second student in this placement, I benefited from the fact that the team had a good understanding of the potential for an occupational science focus and they suggested 'Futures' as an appropriate area for my involvement as my placement coincided with the commencement of the course. This meant that I was able to experience the 'Futures' course in totality; however, I was unable to have any influence on the course structure or content as this had already been decided by the team following the preliminary work carried out by Philippa. Being the second student in a role emerging setting was simultaneously daunting and encouraging; I understood that the team was receptive but I was also aware that there would be ideas and preconceptions about my skills, abilities and interests and perhaps I would not meet these expectations. Philippa's project provided the context for 'Futures', and assisted me to create a role within the team quickly as the importance of an occupational therapy perspective was immediately apparent. As the only student in my cohort to 'follow in another's footsteps' I had the unique perspective of observing how highly the team valued our 'holistic' viewpoint.

An advantage of the autonomy provided by the role emerging experience was that I was able to identify and negotiate my specific project based on what I felt would be beneficial for the placement and achievable within my timeframe. I initially explored the idea suggested by the Travellers Education Service of developing a project supporting 'Futures' that focused on devising learning pathways for each student, to provide the course with an individualised element. However, it quickly became apparent that this was unrealistic, as building an effective therapeutic relationship would take much longer than the time available. Through the support provided by my practice placement educators I was able to identify that an occupationally focused evaluation of the course would be a more appropriate project. The purpose of this was to provide guidance to assist in future development of the course, identifying strengths and weaknesses from an occupational perspective. I found devising and implementing the evaluation portion of 'Futures' challenging. However, through effective clinical supervision and reflection I realised that without a professional (occupational therapist) lead in the team I had relied on my understanding of an occupational therapist's role in a traditional setting, rather than looking at the wider perspective. Consequently, I became focussed on providing an almost 'clinical' intervention, as this was a role with which I felt familiar and as a result I experienced frustration and diminishing confidence as it became apparent this would not be possible. Whilst I had the knowledge to understand that building a therapeutic relationship and collaborative goals takes time, which was not feasible within the course structure, it took the external guidance provided through supervision, rather than my skill as a therapist, to enable me to recognise this as the limiting factor (Mattingly & Fleming, 1994; Finlay, 2004). Nevertheless, I found that the project was helpful since it required me to maintain my 'occupational' focus, rather than becoming subsumed as another Travellers Education Service staff member in my desire to become a beneficial addition to the team. I now recognise that I became overly focussed on this requirement in the early stages of the placement, and this impeded my creativity in how occupational science can be applied. For example, my evaluation of 'Futures' conceptualised the occupational needs of Gypsy Travellers and assisted the staff by providing another viewpoint on their cultural needs and the issues they face. It highlighted how their course helped to meet these needs, and the areas for further development. This was vital because, whilst the course had some successes, it did not achieve all its aims as the staff did not fully acknowledge why it takes time to assist the students to develop the motivation, interest and confidence to overcome personal and environmental barriers and the importance of making the activities personally meaningful (Finlay, 2004; Kielhofner, 2004). The evaluation of the course was well received, and the staff intended to use the ideas proposed in future courses. For me, this reinforced the value of the placement and promoted my self-confidence in aspects of service development.

Contributing to future practice

The role emerging placement provided invaluable learning opportunities. Apart from promoting professionalism and proficiency in project management, the placement encouraged both students to assess their general understanding of humans as occupational beings. Furthermore, without the exposure to this unique and fascinating client group, neither student would have had the opportunity to consider and question her own sympathies and prejudices regarding Travellers in general.

The role emerging placements described, highlighted to the students the occupational risk factors impacting on Travellers, particularly the young adults in these communities. The students were able to apply their theoretical understanding of occupational science to form an accurate occupational perspective of the individuals with whom they worked. The placements offered them the opportunity to identify and address the occupational needs of the service users and work in an autonomous way to develop core occupational therapy skills.

Although now working in different settings, both students feel that the role emerging placement has provided them with invaluable tools for practice. Philippa currently works in a forensic setting and the role emerging experience made her acutely aware of the impact of occupational risk factors on health and well-being. This experience has also developed her confidence in applying these issues in practice to promote the occupational therapy role and justify interventions. Furthermore, the opportunity to engage in project management and practice development on this placement has subsequently led to greater confidence in her ability to engage in these responsibilities in her current role.

Lydia is currently employed in social services, within a diverse ethnic community. She has found that the role emerging placement has developed her skills in challenging her own prejudices, and is using this to practice in a culturally sensitive manner. Additionally, the experience has assisted her in becoming self-directed in applying theoretical models to conceptualise human occupational behaviour and using this to support clinical interventions.

Elisha's Canadian experience

Professional practice placements are, by their very nature, intended to be challenging, enriching and replete with the kind of learning that will both prepare students for future practice and enable them to succeed as autonomous clinicians. Each and every placement completed throughout the course of my degree programme fostered new skills and permitted both personal and professional growth, but it was the role emerging placement that allowed me to consolidate two years of intensive learning into my own vision and approach to occupation focused practice.

Setting the stage: occupational therapy in primary health care

Role emerging placements, by design, are inherently innovative and often aptly defined as "out-of-the-box". This line of reasoning can inspire excitement, even curiosity, and also uncertainty, anxiety and tinges of fear, particularly as a student clamouring to acquire every possible ounce of practical skill and proficiency prior to graduation. With two years of schooling drawing to a close and one final, 8-week practicum, expectations for our concluding placement ran high. As a student armed with minimal understanding of the role emerging placement, and no first-hand experience to capitalise on, the notion of entering my last placement in this capacity was unsettling and destabilising – two forces that I would later realise to be indispensable to the learning process. Wood (2005) distinguishes role emerging placements from standard clinical learning by the immersion of student therapists in a non-traditional practice environment that does not employ an occupational therapist and in which supports are provided by an off-site preceptor/mentor. By virtue of this fact, formulation of a distinct occupational therapy role is often in its infancy, if at all established, and the structure of such a position remains somewhat ill defined and protean. Despite its situation within a busy Family Health Team (FHT) with no formally established occupational therapy service, this particular role emerging placement was under girded by a strong vision of occupational therapy and rehabilitation within primary health care and compelling initial evidence to suggest both fit and effectiveness in this setting. Building upon earlier efforts to increase the presence of rehabilitation services within primary care, this practicum benefited from the lessons gleaned by previous researchers and students who had laid the groundwork for this challenging placement.

Family Health Teams (FHT) are one component of the Ontario government's strategy to improve health access and quality for consumers. These teams are designed to function as a coordinated suite of interdisciplinary services, capable of providing comprehensive primary care to a discrete population (Ministry of Health and Long-Term Care, 2009). Explicit in this model is an emphasis on comprehensive, holistic care comprised of not only direct service provision, but health promotion, disease/disability prevention and chronic disease management (HealthForceOntario, 2009). Central to this placement was a population-based approach to health and the delivery of a rehabilitation-focused chronic disease self-management group programme, offered in conjunction with individualised, one-on-one service provision and support. In keeping with the tenets of collaborative, interdisciplinary primary care, this placement was carried out in partnership with a student physical therapist and precepted by supervisors from both disciplines. As students, we were on site daily and worked in close cooperation not only with nursing and physician services but also several allied health professions, including social work, nutrition and pharmacy. Service delivery was premised primarily on a direct model of care, but incorporated aspects of a consultative approach as well. Multiple non-clinical staff members assisted in various aspects of placement coordination and logistics, orientation, student education and induction. It was this combination of clinical and non-clinical supports that proved to be instrumental to both the efficiency and success of the practicum experience.

Historically, and by definition, role emerging placements often flow from settings in which no occupational therapy role has been identified or established (Thew et al., 2008). While this may be true of my placement to some degree, the natural compatibility of occupational therapy and primary health care had already generated interest within the FHT and broader community as a result of earlier students and ongoing research to support the evidence base for rehabilitation in such settings. This is not to imply that the placement was without pitfalls, but to underscore the fact that select key stakeholders had already embraced the notion of rehabilitation as a component of primary health care in the FHT.

The formidable task presented to us was to create a programme with the buy-in of team members and the patients/clients they cared for. In order to launch a sustainable and relevant programme, it was essential to convey an image of occupational therapy that was reflective of the professions core values and beliefs and consistent with the services being provided. Compounding this challenge was the need to clearly differentiate my occupational therapist role and competencies from those of physiotherapy and my student counterpart and collaborator. Many FHT staff demonstrated a basic understanding of the profession, but few were able to perceive of occupational therapy's potential role within the broader picture of primary care. Because occupational therapy is so often misunderstood, it was essential to capture the functional, occupation-focused spirit of our services. In addition to daily service delivery, the use of concrete examples and case scenarios, coupled with marketing and educational materials, staff communication bulletins and "teaching moments" proved to be the most fruitful means of heightening occupational therapy's profile within the clinic. Inter-professional collaboration through workshops and internal referrals acted to not only raise the staff and clients' awareness of occupational therapy, but also the complementary inter-relationships between disciplines. Once staff was better equipped to grasp the occupational nature of this role, connections between occupation, health and well-being fell into place. As a role emerging placement, this setting naturally supported occupation-based practice because it was not hemmed in by a pre-supposed framework and could be reshaped as the complexities and nuances unfolded.

Role development necessitated that we carve out a niche distinct enough to separate us from other disciplines, yet congruent enough to demonstrate overall fit within the team. In line with the philosophy of primary health care, the goal of this programme was to promote health and prevent disability by enabling occupational functioning and reducing barriers to participation. The focus on function allowed both occupational and physical therapy to deliver services in a harmonious manner, while still respecting the individuality of the respective professions and ensuring that referrals were diverted to the appropriate team member. While this inter-professional model of the role emerging placement did present some initial challenges, it fostered sound role delineation for both me as a student, and for the staff and clients to whom we were targeting our services. Working intimately with a student physical therapist encouraged me to further my appreciation of their profession and to expand my clinical skill set within domains that are not always within the purview of occupational therapy. For our clients, inter-professional assessment and intervention often meant the merging of two distinct bodies of knowledge working towards one shared goal. The opportunity to eke out our own role and collaborate with complementary disciplines opened my eyes to facets of occupational therapy that I did not realise existed, or that I was once reluctant to explore. Examples of such interdisciplinary partnering abound and ranged from joint PT/OT exercise counselling and environmental barrier identification to group pain management offered in conjunction with social work, nutrition and pharmacy.

Both group and individual sessions were offered either jointly with occupational and physical therapy students or one-on-one as appropriate. Client-centred practice, with critical emphasis on individualised goal setting, encouraged clients to dictate the performance issues addressed and ranged from home visits and environmental assessments to functional mobility evaluation, community participation, exercise counselling, energy conservation, assistive device prescription, cognitive and behavioural strategies, community referral and coordination, splinting, education, meaningful activity and pain management to name a few. In addition, an evidence-based weekly chronic disease rehabilitation self-management programme was delivered in collaboration with supervisors from both occupational and physical therapy. All assessments and interventions were documented electronically, in order to maximise the integration of services and to provide physicians with ongoing progress reports.

The transience of occupational therapy's presence (i.e. service was limited to student placement periods and associated research endeavours) and high medical resident turnover within the clinic posed certain barriers to referral generation and determination of the populations occupational needs. Once our programme's direction and intended role were communicated to practitioners within the FHT, the task of securing clients assumed paramount importance. In addition to marketing efforts undertaken within the clinic and among staff, physician and allied health screening and recruitment became increasingly important. Occupational needs were determined by both referring clinicians and the clients themselves, and expanded upon gaps identified by previous student placements and research endeavours. Although being a time-limited programme based on the eight-week duration of our placement, as student therapists we made ourselves available to clients as intensively as they required and in a variety of environments (e.g. home, gym and clinic). Direct service provision was further supplemented by consultative practices, with additional rehabilitation input, screening and resources provided to other allied health practitioners and physicians in person and electronically. Programme effectiveness and outcomes were evaluated through several indicators, including client self-report, participation/uptake, referral tracking and surveys. Persistent need for further student placements and continued patient requests for both occupational and physical therapy are evidence that such services met an identified need and have a place within this primary care setting.

Change is often slow to come and difficult to sustain. Entering into a role emerging placement, with no guarantee of programme continuity, we were acutely aware of the need for capacity building and measures to ensure carry-over for clients. Attempts to promote the sustainability of both the occupational and physical therapy programmes were made through the creation of a programme manual and resource collection for prospective students. Detailed caseload and wait lists were maintained to assist future students with referral generation and the opportunity to carry forward client goals and plans as set out with previous student therapists. In the spirit of the self-management programmes taught, goal-setting and action-planning skills were introduced and reinforced as a means of sustaining progress, even without an ever-present rehabilitation programme. A myriad of factors can be cited in the overall success of this learning process. The fruitfulness of my experience as a student in a non-traditional, role emerging practicum was contoured by everything from the model of supervision and student education, to the degree of structure imposed, community/clinic attitudes and perceptions, placement preparation and planning, method of evaluation and level of clinical experience. Inter-professional student collaboration and joint mentorship/supervision by both occupational and physical therapists stressed peer support and interdisciplinary learning, while heightening insight into the similarities, differences and overlap of professions. As a result of preliminary placements at the site and ongoing research, programme development and role identification was shaped by a delicate balance of both pre-existing conceptualisations and the freedom to expand and adapt as needed. The absence of policy, protocol and a standardised approach to service delivery presented challenges at times, but encouraged us to think creatively and critically, to question and justify the logic behind our reasoning and behaviours and to practice in a manner consistent with what occupational therapy meant to me. As a student, everyday situations and dilemmas required me to evaluate the lens through which I was viewing the world and helped bridge theory to practice, a process that was facilitated through journaling and weekly communication with preceptors. The autonomy of this placement and a modest set of clinical skills and experience to draw on necessitated self-direction and the operationalisation of evidence-based, reflective practice.

In preparing for and engaging in this practicum experience, it was readily apparent how instrumental staff and client sentiment, attitude and perception were to the learning outcomes. As a whole, staff was widely receptive to the notion of rehabilitation services within the primary care setting, a fact evidenced by interdisciplinary referrals, collaborative education sessions, willingness to accommodate new service demands and the sense of value conferred upon our programmes. Legitimising this role to key stakeholders required that staff understood both the intent and focus of the programmes, and that communication was not simply a rote exercise but a daily expectation. Physical space to operate our programmes, though seemingly less important than mentality, was key to our ability to provide a reliable service to new clients. Within this model of student education, reduced access to supervisors and fewer opportunities to evaluate learning behaviours demanded that expectations and objectives were clearly set out and adaptable enough to evolve with the role itself. The readiness of preceptors to provide mentorship within this non-traditional model cannot be overlooked as a decisive factor in the success of this type of fieldwork. Exposure to an array of clinical settings and level of student experience must be considered when matching students with roles in which there is no formally established service or programme, as I would not have possessed the basic repertoire of skills on which such a placement is premised as a novice student.

Fieldwork education is an indispensable tool in the clinical learning process (Bossers et al., 1997). Each successive placement as a student therapist helped to prepare me for practice in distinct ways, imparting lessons that I have carried forward since entering practice. Communication, rapport building, critical thinking, self-directedness, clinical reasoning, programme development, needs assessment, professional advocacy, reflective practice and comfort with change and uncertainty are skills that may proceed from many placements but that were consolidated as a student confronted with the complexities of role emerging practice. A substantial body of literature has demonstrated the inextricable link between positive health outcomes and the delivery of evidence-based occupational therapy services within a multitude of primary care settings (Klaiman, 2004; Canadian Association of Occupational Therapists, 2006). Nevertheless, calls to increase access to appropriate services and expand the role of rehabilitation in primary health care have fallen short and efforts to further demonstrate the utility of occupational therapy in such settings will continue to be the impetus for similar role emerging placements. To this day, research and student placements remain a fixture within this busy, primary care clinic – a rallying cry of sorts, aimed at maintaining these breakthroughs and new boundaries of practice. On a personal note, what is more telling or indicative of the need for occupational therapy services, than to recognise the names of my former clients, still crossing the desk of new students, two years later.

While no single placement can prepare you entirely for practice, each leaves an indelible mark. My REP experience was not without challenges, but it ultimately equipped me with the transferable skills of self-direction, critical thinking and curiosity. As a relatively new graduate, I have worked in a variety of practice settings, from community to hospital-based care, each time entering a new environment with the confidence to approach practice in a manner consistent with my values and occupation-centred beliefs. As a clinician, I believe strongly in my role and the value of occupation – and it was through the REP experience that the importance of advocacy, on behalf of our clients and profession, became engrained.

Conclusion

This chapter has provided the perspective of three student occupational therapists engaged in role emerging practice situations. Challenges encountered and lessons learned have been shared. While the practice settings were different, common issues arose. The importance of establishing realistic expectations for student involvement/projects is key to the success of the learning experience. Developing legacy material for subsequent students to build upon helps refine and consolidate the learning, educate current interdisciplinary team members and assist with ensuring that student occupational therapists are adding an occupational perspective to the team initiatives and are not just providing 'an additional pair of hands'. Although traditional occupational therapy placements promote clinical experience, role emerging placements offer opportunities to encourage independence, validate learning and support confidence in practice. The role emerging placement is an opportunity to understand how occupational science and the tenets central to the discipline can benefit practice by incorporating them through creative working and using the therapists' skills and clinical reasoning. A role emerging placement is a fantastic opportunity to fully appreciate what skills an occupational therapist has, without relying on an established role or way of working. This in turn can encourage clinicians to expand their role outside conventional settings to support the expansion of occupational therapy as a profession and establish ways to promote the value of occupational therapy intervention.

References

Bancroft, A, Llyod, M, & Morran, R. (1996). *The Right to Roam – Travellers in Scotland 1995/69.* Dunfermline: Save the Children Fund.

Bossers, A., Cook, J., Polatajko, H., & Laine, C. (1997). Understanding the role-emerging fieldwork placement. *Canadian Journal of Occupational Therapy, 64,* 70–81.

Canadian Association of Occupational Therapists. (2006). Canadian Association of Occupational Therapists position statement: Occupational therapy and primary health care. *Canadian Journal of Occupational Therapists, 73,* 122–123.

Daniels, N. (2007). Practice placement supervision models. *OT News, 15* (7), 23.

Derrington, C., & Kendall, S. (2004). *Gypsy Traveller Students in Secondary Schools: Cultural identity and Achievement.* Stoke on Trent: Trentham Books.

Every Traveller Child Matters. (2007). *Liverpool Traveller Education Service.* Every Child Matters Handbook.

Finlay, L. (2004) *The Practice of Psychosocial Occupational Therapy* (3rd ed.). London: Nelson Thornes.

Goward. P, Repper. Appleton, L., & Hagan, T. (2006). Crossing boundaries. Identifying and meeting the mental health needs of gypsies and travellers. *Journal of Mental Health, 15* (3), 315–327.

HealthForceOntario. (2009). *Primary Health Care.* Retrieved 9 August 2009, from http://www.healthforceontario.ca/HealthcareInOntario/PrimaryCare.aspx.

Klaiman, D. (2004). Increasing access to occupational therapy in primary health care. *OT Now, 6,* 14–19.

Kielhofner, G. (2004). *Conceptual Foundations of Occupational Therapy* (3rd ed.). Philadelphia: F.A. Davis.

Lomax, D, Lancaster, S, & Gray, P. (2000). *Moving on: A Survey of Travellers' Views.* Edinburgh: The Scottish Executive Central Research Unit.

Mattingly, C., & Fleming, M.H. (1994). *Clinical reasoning Forms of Inquiry in a Therapeutic Practice.* Philadelphia, F.A. Davis.

Minato, M., & Zemke, R. (2004). Occupational choices of persons with schizophrenia living in the community. *Journal of Occupational Science, 11* (1), 31–39.

Ministry of Health and Long-Term Care. (2009). Family health teams: Your access to primary health care. Retrieved 9 August 2009, from http://www.health.gov.on.ca/transformation/fht/fht_mn.html.

Race Relations Act. (1976). *c.74.* London: HMSO.

Thew, M., Hargreaves, A., & Cronin-Davis, J. (2008). An evaluation of a role-emerging practice placement model for a full cohort of occupational therapy students. *British Journal of Occupational Therapy. 71* (8), 348–353.

Wilcock, A. (1998). *An Occupational Perspective of Health* (2nd ed.). Thorofare, New Jersey: SLACK Inc.

Wilcock, A, & Townsend, E. (2000). Occupational terminology interactive dialogue: Occupational justice. *Journal of Occupational Science, 7* (2), 84–86.

Wood, A. (2005). Student practice contexts: Changing face, changing place. *British Journal of Occupational Therapy. 68* (8), 375–378.

Chapter 5

Promoting well-being in a large organisation: Challenges and opportunities

Miranda Thew

Introduction

Well-being is considered to be related to the subjective measurement of overall happiness and/or satisfaction with life, which can be influenced by wealth, health, personality and by what we do or engage in (Argyle, 2001; Diener et al., 2003; Eid & Larsen, 2008). Ryan and Deci (2001) more succinctly describe well-being as "optimal psychological functioning and experience" (p. 142). What is clear is that health is often seen to be synonymous with the human state of well-being. If ill-health is being experienced it is likely that subjective well-being will be influenced, evidence suggests that satisfaction with life and a poor sense of well-being can also precipitate ill-health or lead to poorer prognosis in disease (Groenvold et al., 2007). Working-age adults are said to spend on average between 40 hours (males) and 26 hours (females) per week occupied by paid work (Aguiar & Hurst, 2007). Paid work has already been acknowledged as being an essential contributing factor in the health and well-being of working-age adults. These factors are considerably more than that of financial reward or the status that a job can bring. The workplace is considered a major setting which can make a difference in terms of actively enhancing well-being, and therefore in promoting health and preventing ill health (Kreis & Bödeker, 2004; Rahtz & Szykman 2008). However, there are instances where the workplace can contribute to ill-health, for example, in the case of work-related stress (Health and Safety Executive, 2007). This has led to many employers to have a vested interest in economic but effective work-based health promotion programmes. Such programmes can make an impact, particularly in encouraging healthier diets and increased amounts of exercise (Pelletier, 2005). This chapter reflects the growing emphasis by national and international health drivers on employers to take more responsibility towards staff health and well-being and not just when illness strikes.

Occupational therapists have already established themselves in vocational rehabilitation or return to work programmes particularly for those facing some form of disability (Ross, 2007). However, few have actively engaged or disseminated their experience of developing well-being within an essentially well population of employees. This chapter explores the experience of one occupational therapist in contributing to enhancing well-being for staff working within a large Higher Education Institution (HEI) in the United Kingdom (UK).

Role Emerging Occupational Therapy: Maximising Occupation-Focused Practice, 1st edition. Edited by Miranda Thew, Mary Edwards, Sue Baptiste and Matthew Molineux. © 2011 Blackwell Publishing Ltd.

This includes preventing and addressing workplace stress, and managing lifestyle issues such as fatigue, retirement and occupational balance. By describing the experience of an occupational therapist and the use of lifestyle management strategies to enhance well-being it is hoped that other occupational therapists could consider and value this kind of health promotion role within essentially healthy populations in the workplace.

The current 'climate' in healthy lifestyles and well-being

Currently the health agenda of the UK like many western nations is particularly focussed on promoting health and healthy lifestyles (DoH, 2004). Health promoting research and activity has grown exponentially in the past decade, especially within well yet 'vulnerable' populations. This is supported by the increasing evidence that personal lifestyles can influence the severity and timing of long-term morbidity and premature mortality (Chiuve et al., 2006; Dantzer et al., 2006; Kurth et al., 2006). Coronary heart disease (CHD), for example, causes the highest rate of all adult deaths in the UK (in keeping with most affluent nations); of those, 20% of CHD deaths in men and 17% in women are attributable to lifestyle (World Health Organization (WHO), 2002). Feeling satisfied with life and not feeling adversely stressed has been correlated with greater recovery time from physical illness and disease, conversely, low mood and stress has been associated with increased likelihood of death from cancer, CHD and other major diseases (Colton & Manderschied, 2006; Siahpush et al., 2008).

The occupations people choose to engage in can to a lesser or greater extent influence lifestyles (Velde and Fidler, 2002; Christiansen & Townsend, 2004; Hammel, 2004). How people view their daily occupations in terms of meaning and significance and the relevance to well-being are factors that occupational scientists and occupational therapists are particularly well suited to understand and address (Christiansen & Matuska, 2006). Wilcock (1998) offers some clear direction in how to view occupation and health or well-being. Her view has been more recently illustrated in Figure 5.1. In essence, she

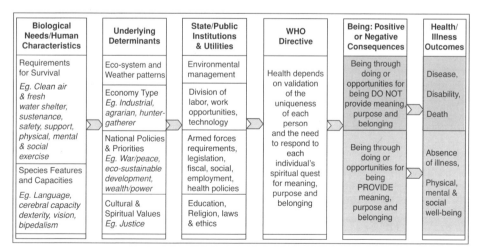

Biological Needs/Human Characteristics	Underlying Determinants	State/Public Institutions & Utilities	WHO Directive	Being: Positive or Negative Consequences	Health/ Illness Outcomes
Requirements for Survival *Eg. Clean air & fresh water shelter, sustenance, safety, support, physical, mental & social exercise* Species Features and Capacities *Eg. Language, cerebral capacity dexterity, vision, bipedalism*	Eco-system and Weather patterns Economy Type *Eg. Industrial, agrarian, hunter-gatherer* National Policies & Priorities *Eg. War/peace, eco-sustainable development, wealth/power* Cultural & Spiritual Values *Eg. Justice*	Environmental management Division of labor, work opportunities, technology Armed forces requirements, legislation, fiscal, social, employment, health policies Education, Religion, laws & ethics	Health depends on validation of the uniqueness of each person and the need to respond to each individual's spiritual quest for meaning, purpose and belonging	Being through doing or opportunities for being DO NOT provide meaning, purpose and belonging Being through doing or opportunities for being PROVIDE meaning, purpose and belonging	Disease, Disability, Death Absence of illness, Physical, mental & social well-being

Figure 5.1   Determinants of illness or well-being of being through doing. Wilcock (2006)

builds up the case for self-value to be considered within an individual's innate 'doing' of occupations. Wilcock (2006, p. 6) asserts that "it is only by what they do that people can demonstrate who they are and what they hope to be". She postulates that each person is unique through their choice and engagement in occupation, and that the desire to 'do' is powerful enough to mediate illness and/or overcome the effects of disability. In this respect, well-being is achieved by purposeful and meaningful occupation that reflects a person's inner self, desires, personality and skills. Wilcock also considers that through engagement in meaningful occupation, healthy individuals can maintain their health and well-being and that when deprived of that occupation, then ill-health and poorer satisfaction with life will inevitably follow. To many working-age adults the single most influential occupation will be the one in which they spend most time, this clearly should therefore be of particular resonance within occupational science and occupational therapy.

The importance of work as an occupation

Many working-age adults proportionally occupy more of their time in paid work than engaged in any other single occupation, and this is particularly so in the UK (Aguiar & Hurst, 2007; Chatzitheochari and Arber, 2009). Literature suggests that being employed is associated with a greater sense of self-esteem, improved health, higher socio-economic status and longevity (Gerdtham & Johannesson, 2003; Creed & Macintyre, 2001). Waddell and Burton's (2006) review of the evidence regarding the relationship between work, health and well-being concluded that "work is overall generally good for health and well-being ... the beneficial effects of work outweigh the risks of work and are greater than the harmful effects of long-term unemployment and long-term sickness absence" (p. ix). Although their extensive appraisal of literature recognises the influence of employment in people's health status, they also caution that the nature, quality and social context of paid work can have detrimental effects. But more importantly, work is considered to support human volition and identity, in that being productive can foster a sense of self-achievement and fulfilment, which is key to self-esteem and personal motivation, as well as providing an identifiable role that is paid for and therefore is valued (Kielhofner, 2002).

Studies suggest that investment in return to work programmes and supported work placements can pay dividends to recovery and improvement in long-term outcomes to illness and disease (Catty et al., 2008; Burns et al., 2009). Occupational therapy interventions in return to work have been recognised as being beneficial in the improvement of their condition such as depression (de Vries & Schene, 2009). Even when there are barriers to being at work through disability, many people desire to continue to work despite frequently facing problems in being able to enjoy, thrive and be successful in staying within the work-place (Roulstone, 2003). Given the importance therefore, of being in work in maintaining, contributing and supporting health and well-being, it is highly relevant that worksites are important public health/health promotion settings (Linnan et al., 2008). WHO (1995) suggested that the health of human beings within the world could be enhanced via the institutions and places in which people work. The UK government has already taken steps to change work and leisure environments with such policies as the ban on smoking in public areas and places of employment (DoH, 2006). In the UK government's 'Choosing Health' white paper the emphasis is on encouraging employers to take more responsibility for employee health and create settings to promote health and well-being (DoH, 2004). There are also moves by the government to reform the manner in which people are managed when they are absent from work due to sickness (Black, 2008). What is also emerging is that early or premature retirement is associated with having experienced poor mental health, unfavourable working conditions and work vs. family conflicts whilst at work (Aromaa & Koskinen, 2002).

One of the fundamental issues influencing the health of workers is job satisfaction; employees attribute nearly a quarter of their life satisfaction to job happiness (Faragher et al., 2005; Grawitch et al., 2007). Job satisfaction has been found to be so strongly associated with mental/psychological problems that dissatisfaction at work could be considered hazardous to an employee's mental health and well-being (Faragher et al., 2005). Those who most often reported 'job strain' had a higher incidence of medical conditions including high blood pressure, heart disease and diabetes (Carroll et al., 2001). Wellness at work can also be influenced by the type of 'spill-over' (i.e. the effect that a bad day at work can spill-over into home or vice versa) (McKenna & Thew, 2008). Positive spill-over from work-to-home has been associated with better physical and mental health; conversely, if that spill-over is negative, there are associations with poorer physical and mental health (Grzywacz & Marks, 2000).

Keeping people at work is an important national governmental driver. The cost to the UK economy of people not working due to illness has been estimated at being over £100 billion per year (Black, 2008). It is a widely accepted fact that the longer an individual remains off work, the more difficult return to work becomes, with subsequent economic and social deprivation (Henderson et al., 2005). Indeed, only 20% of people receiving incapacity benefit for more than six months will return to work in the following five years (Department for Work and Pensions, 2002). Two million people suffer an illness that they believe has been caused, or has been made worse, by their job (Department of Health (DoH), 2004). An example of a large employer where potentially staff are at risk of absences due to ill health is the National Health Service (NHS) itself, The Wanless (2004) report suggested that the NHS has large employee sickness levels (costing an estimated £1 billion a year), yet, lacked formal work-based preventative strategies or programmes. Mental health problems are a leading cause of absenteeism from paid work (WHO, 2005; Black, 2008). There has been a range of workplace policies and interventions developed across Europe promoting positive understanding and enabling people to remain in the workforce with a mental health problem (Curran et al., 2007). Indeed, within HEIs the major cause of illness and sickness absence in academic staff is mental health or psycho-social problems, predominantly stress-related (Houston et al., 2006; Kinman, 2008). Physical illnesses and musculoskeletal problems, which are much more common in manufacturing or construction work environments, are largely confined at HEIs to support services staff, such as porters, security officers and cleaners (Kumar & Kumar, 2008). Tytherleigh et al. (2005) conclude that the multiple changes within the UK higher education sector and lack of control in work roles are also contributing to high levels of stress. This tends to suggest that interventions in the workplace are needed to address the psycho-social factors that can influence well-being.

Within the UK, employers have been given support and guidance towards recognising work-based stress as being a hazard to employee's health (Health and Safety Executive,

2003). The Health and Safety Executive (HSE) can use health and safety law to steer companies to taking 'reasonable' steps to prevent exposing employees to unreasonable levels of pressure at work. However, their main role is to provide advice to enable managers to consider certain risk factors within the workplace which are said to contribute to work-related stress. Six management standards have been recommended which are essentially good management practices (HSE, 2005). Each employer has to demonstrate that they are actively pursuing the practice of these management standards and measuring and assessing work-based stress risk. The HSE places the emphasis on the employers and on prevention, but what is particularly worrying is the lack of services that can help people with work-related or other situational stress. The National Institute of Clinical Excellence (NICE) recommends that people experiencing significant stress should receive appropriate interventions (NICE, 2004), however, GPs are unable to refer to them because there are not enough staff available who are suitably trained or experienced (Layard, 2005). Stress management is an important element within the range of therapeutic skills that occupational therapists use within a variety of contexts, particularly within the psychosocial paradigms of health (Stein & Cutler, 2002). Occupational therapists are also key professionals in lifestyle management advice (Clark et al., 1997; Mountain et al., 2008; Thew & McKenna, 2008). Encouraging participation in meaningful occupations outside of work may prove a valuable, but informal, stress reduction strategy (Zuzanek, 1998). Studies have proven the effectiveness of occupational therapy in improving the quality of lives and preventing ill-health in well populations (Clarke et al, 1997, Mountain et al., 2008). There are few other professions that have the understanding of person, occupations and the environment, and conceptualising or supporting the dynamic balance between those components (Hagedorn, 2000; Law & Baum, 2005). However, the profession of occupational therapy has been traditionally focussed on measuring and improving or enabling occupational performance once illness or disability strikes (Whiteford et al., 2005). This is reflected in return to paid or non-paid work following illness or disability has historically been a key role for occupational therapists for many years (Holmes, 2007; Ross, 2007). That said, occupational therapists in the UK who work in vocational rehabilitation do so within clinical and statutory settings (such as the NHS), they are rarely found within the private or occupational health sector (Holmes, 2007). There many examples are of international drivers that encompass the importance of engaging with occupations and the links to health (Wilcock, 2006). Yet, there is a lack of awareness that the expertise of an occupational therapist, with their 'holistic' professional training encompassing mental and physical health and social care could be a potentially potent asset within an occupational health paradigm (Wilcock, 2005; Stein & Cutler, 2002).

Worksite well-being programmes

The costs to an organisation not only in terms of decreased productivity but also the effect on others of carrying an extra workload when someone is absent from work has led to many organisations developing well-being and health-promotion programmes to prevent sickness absence (Kreis & Bödeker, 2004; Rahtz & Szykman 2008). Moreover, Anand-Keller et al. (2009) suggest not only costs benefits to the organisation in providing staff programmes but also in terms of a moral duty of the employer, as well as reducing the cost to national health services. Despite such programmes considered to be a worthwhile investment to large employers (Bertera, 1990; Goetzel et al., 2004; Pelletier et al., 2004), it appears, that the companies investing are mainly from the private sector, particularly in countries where health insurance covers the costs (Childress & Lindsay, 2006). Programmes for staff have proved effective in changing lifestyle behaviours and in return to work (Goetzel et al., 2002; Cook et al., 2007; Salmi et al., 2009). If well-being interventions are interactive, 'tailor made' to meet the needs of the employees, and evidence based, there is evidence that they can enhance employee health and quality of life, and still provide a cost reduction to the employer (Arnand-Keller et al., 2009; Burke, 2009). Moreover, if well-being programmes are supported and attended by senior managers, based on sound cognitive-behavioural principles and led by experienced qualified staff, the success of a well-being programme also increases (Goetzel & Ozminkowski, 2008).

WHO (1995) recognises the important roles that the field of occupational health and health and safety teams have in promoting health and preventing injury or harm from work. However, it also supports initiatives and 'experts' from other areas to support these teams. An occupational therapist has an important role potentially here; however, it appears that many occupational therapists are not fully conversant with current health and safety law, possibly due to a lack of emphasis in occupational therapy pre-registration training (Ross, 2007). There is a dearth of evidence suggesting a role for occupational therapists directly working as part of an occupational health team. This presents a missed opportunity, especially in the current climate with heightened emphasis on addressing health risks at work, the latest and most noteworthy, being the risk of stress in the work place (HSE, 2003). This development from the HSE offers potential roles for therapists, as they are constantly assessing the risk to health through engagement in occupations (Clemson et al., 1999; Hughes, 2008; Clemson, 2009). If more occupational therapists could look beyond their roles of being mainly restricted to vocational rehabilitation they may recognise the valuable contribution they could make within occupational health and well-being. As it currently stands, occupational health teams predominantly consist of mainly nurses or physicians. The overall aim of occupational health nurses is to 'achieve improvements in the health of working people' (Oakley, 2002, p. 1). Typically, but not exclusively, these are nurses with specialist advanced education who work closely alongside health and safety staff and, in particular, offer advice on employees' return to work following absence, retaining staff at the workplace and work/health-related hazards (WHO, 2001). They are also directly involved in health promotion programmes however; many feel that they are not able to devote as much time to promoting health and well-being due to resources and demands on more traditional tasks and roles (Mellor & St John, 2007) offering yet more opportunity to occupational therapists.

An example of a occupational therapists contribution

Given the current emphasis on lifestyles and health promotion, well-being, stress as a work hazard, and the desire to keep people at work when facing illness and disability, the role of an occupational therapist is quite obvious. However, the first issue to overcome is the fact that an occupational therapist's role and the understanding of the profession is not well known especially outside of the health care field. One of the principle ways 'in' to having the skills of an occupational therapist recognised by others is by practically demonstrating how an occupational therapist can make a difference to staff well-being at work. This was achieved in this example, by offering to facilitate several sessions to the staff development programme. This then led to recognition by senior managers in the university that there was a 'local' in house expert in addressing issues of stress and well-being within the university, a secondment opportunity then arose to specifically address the risk of work-related stress. However, this role soon allowed for a more diverse range of strategies to be developed; these included:

1) University managers' stress risk assessment training;
2) the development and facilitation of a stress and lifestyle management group;
3) the contribution to the development and content of a university well-being website;
4) provision of occupation focused interventions on a healthy retirement programme for staff.

1) University managers' stress risk assessment training.

This was a mandatory (including corporate level) managers' training workshop which was devised conjointly with a senior manager of safety, health and well-being; the material on stress risk assessment was centred largely around the six HSE (2003) management standards already mentioned. The occupational therapist in this example, enhanced the material by providing an insight as to how workplace stress can be recognised, and demonstrated a range of techniques and strategies to help build resilience to stress and thereby maximise occupational performance at work (Box 5.1). There were joint presentations on how managers can develop 'psychologically healthy' work environments, with an emphasis on trying to educate people regarding the effects of stress on lifestyles and vice versa. The mandatory nature of the training package for all managers across the university added an aspect of ensuring that key aspects such as occupational balance and meaningful occupation were made cognisant. Managers could also opt for an enhanced day-long session that incorporated an even greater range of personal coping strategies all of which were devised by an occupational therapist.

2) The development and facilitation of a staff stress and lifestyle management group.

This group was facilitated by two qualified health professionals; an occupational therapist and an occupational health nurse. Most of the material was devised and designed by the occupational therapist, and the content reflected her many years specialising in stress and

---

Box 5.1:   Occupational therapist's contribution to university managers' stress risk assessment training

i) Recognising the causes of stress (e.g. meaningless occupation).
ii) Teaching of portable relaxation strategies which can be applied to enhance occupational performance (Thew, 2008).
iii) Understanding occupational balance (McKenna & Thew, 2008).
iv) Developing insight into the factors of lifestyle that can undermine health (Thew & McKenna, 2008).

Table 5.1   Stress and lifestyle management course content.

Week/Theme	Content
1) Introduction: What is stress?	What is stress? Lifestyle issues. Physiological effects/link to long-term illness. Portable relaxation (Thew, 2008a). Goal setting: identify, re-introduce/engage in one relaxing, meaningful occupation.
2) Understanding causes of lifestyle and stress problems	Lifestyle diaries. Causes of stress. Self report questionnaires. Exploring stress and negative thoughts. Imagery and cognitive relaxation techniques.
3) Managing Sleep and fatigue	Lifestyle diaries. Sleep diaries. Sleep 'hygiene' techniques (Thew, 2008b). Jug of life (Thew & Pemberton, 2008). Fatigue: grading and pacing occupations. Adapting occupations to allow for balanced lifestyle.
4) Communication and relationships!	Examining diaries. Adjusting to change. Relationships. Communicating effectively. Assertiveness techniques. Work colleagues/team working effectiveness.
5) Occupational balance	Understanding concept of balanced occupations in terms of productivity/rest/leisure/personal care. Pleasure = relaxation philosophy. Creating or re-establishing hobbies/meaningful occupations to re-create identities/achievement/promote relaxation.
6) Finish the old, continuing the new	Addressing barriers to change, one sense concentration relaxation techniques. Reviewing diaries. Making changes that last. Goal setting for the future. Evaluate. Complete HAD (Zigmond & Snaith, 1983)

fatigue management within a variety of clinical settings (Table 5.1). All material was evidence based, and the 'pack' of PowerPoint slides, session plans, group activities and handouts can be used commercially for future enterprise revenue for the university. To have such groups supported and promoted by the university is again recognising that stress is real and not simply perceived, and that debilitating symptoms can be managed in order to promote healthier workplace that keep people at work. Each session has handouts/goal setting 'home-work' that relates the experience in group to changes lifestyles and negative cognitions (thoughts/ beliefs). The sessions included the following aspects:

- Occupational balance was taught and supported by handouts and exercises which involved the group members drawing a 'lifestyle circle' (Thew & McKenna, 2008, pp. 61–62). The members were encouraged to divide up the circle according to the different occupations that they spent their time in (the circle as a whole represented a full week of waking hours). However, more significantly, they were asked to highlight and identify the consequential segments according to the emotions and *quality* of the time spent in each occupation. This is particularly relevant in understanding lifestyle balance (Matuska & Christiansen, 2009).

- Time use and lifestyle diaries (specifically that of Thew & Pemberton, 2008, p. 127) allows for analysis of how a person spends their time which is an essential component of an occupational therapists repertoire of assessment skills (Hagedorn, 2001; Matuska & Christiansen, 2009). It allows a person to discover what elements of their lives need change or adaption to free up time for leisure, for example, or to recognise that life is lacking purposeful and meaningful occupation and therefore can negatively influence health.
- Identifying and enhancing meaningful occupation: after using the time use and lifestyle diaries, it could be possible to break those occupations down into lists that indicate those which drain energy, provide energy, are pleasurable or are meaningless (Thew & Pemberton, 2008). This can then be discussed as to what makes the particular occupation draining or meaningless, often this is due to pressure on time and a sense of putting others, such as children's needs above ones own (Craig, 2006).
- Teaching grading and pacing occupations to maximise performance and minimise fatigue and stress: this encompasses a variety of strategies that illustrate how to overcome barriers to engagement to occupations by teaching grading techniques etc. For example, teaching how to pace daily occupations to avoid spending excessive amounts of energy.

Naturally, all the sessions reflected the needs of the group as a whole, and at times, emphasis on a particular element would be necessary; what is clear, is that a 'therapeutic group' is perfectly feasible within the workplace. The groups were particularly well attended; the managers of staff in the group were either recommending the course to their teams or allowed the staff to take time within their working day to attend, the group had been positively promoted by senior managers and in the stress risk assessment material. It was seen by the university to be a positive learning opportunity as opposed to a negative indication of someone's abilities to cope with stress, although it has to be said that this was not measured.

3) Introduction of a university-wide well-being website.

Promotion of health and well-being via the net or a website has been a popular and effective method in which to target populations with advice and support, for example, in weight loss programmes (Booth et al., 2008; Neville et al., 2009), exercise (Spitteals et al., 2007), and stress/depression management (Griffiths & Christiansen, 2006; van Straten et al., 2008). The workplace often provides access to computers and chance to offer tailored advice and support to promote health and improve well-being. However, there have been critics, suggesting that such websites are limited to pamphlets and semi-professional advice (Simpson et al., 2000).

The well-being website in this instance, was predominantly devised and designed by a web designer, a well-being human resources consultant, a Health, Safety and Well-being Manager and an occupational therapist, and had contributions from a variety of staff from across the university. The well-being site opens up by asking the visitor to identify with how they are feeling and what they are thinking about doing. Immediately, the website is considering the person as an occupational being, considering the kinds of occupations (e.g. exams, computer work) that they are participating or wish to participate in. This website not only provides a cohesive hub, directing staff and students to a variety of in-house agencies and to help staff and students successfully manage what they wish to do, but also provides support, advice and strategies to cope with a large range of work related activities. There is advice on work/life balance, time management, fatigue management, insomnia, negative thinking, boredom, inactivity, exercise, healthy eating, relaxation at the computer, etc. All the strategies had to be engaging and available at the fingertips. Self-report questionnaires or tasks to complete for example, a time use diary to recognise occupational imbalance (Mckenna & Thew, 2008) were made available. This cost effective mode of education advice and support not only avoids expensive buying-in of expertise, but allows the website to be commercially viable outside of the university. One important footnote here is that it also provides an opportunity to raise the profile and promote occupational therapy, as in the videos and handouts, there is constant reference (either in introducing the subject or herself) to the profession of occupational therapy. The following specific material was solely devised by the occupational therapist:

i) demonstration of 'portable' relaxation methods (Thew, 2008) with videos (available also on the university You Tube link) and downloadable handouts. These relaxation techniques are useful in that they allow an individual to address symptoms of stress 'in situ' which allows for continued engagement in an occupation. For example, if someone is a teacher and feels extreme stress in controlling a 'difficult' classroom session, a technique such as an abdominal breathing technique, can be followed whilst teaching the class. Occupational therapists focus on maintaining optimal range, choice and performance in occupations (Creek & Lougher, 2008), portable relaxation is just one example of how this is possible.

ii) addressing fatigue and sleep problems; this again involves a video of the techniques and downloadable handouts; these techniques allow an individual to identify (via a 'jug of life and energy' analogy) occupations, relationships and other factors in their life in their life that either drain or provide energy (Thew & Pemberton, 2008. p. 123). This type of analogy along with strategies such as adapting and grading activities, analysing occupations and sleep patterns, getting into life routines and balancing occupations are described and/or demonstrated on the website. All of which are considered to be of particular focus for occupational therapists and which can enable the individual to take control over what they want and need to do (Hagedorn, 2001).

4) Provision of occupation focused interventions on a healthy retirement programme for staff.

Another development opportunity was offered, in terms of offering advice to staff at the university facing retirement. Retirement especially when before the age of 60 has some correlates with premature mortality (Tsai et al., 2005; Dave et al. 2006). The University provides a well-attended two-day programme for staff likely to retire in the next year or so. The sessions are (in the main) facilitated and coordinated by a human resources (HR) consultant, and sessions included looking at pension schemes and financial planning, volunteer opportunities, and stress management. Although stress management was the initial focus requested by the HR team, it was soon obvious by the occupational therapist that issues such as occupational balance and routine as well as encouraging attendees to reflect on meaningful occupation would be more appropriate than learning stress management strategies. There is evidence that if retirees embark on a range of leisure occupations combined with a reduction in work-related stress, that greater health

---

Box 5.2   Content workshop on choosing a relaxing yet meaningful retirement

  i)   Exploring the links between retirement and ill health
 ii)   Links between well-being and occupation
iii)   Group task to identify current meaningful leisure occupations/hobbies
 iv)   Recognition of loss of role and identity that retirement can bring
  v)   Assimilation of link between occupations and well-being and identity
 vi)   Demonstration of relaxation techniques
vii)   Consideration of routines and occupational balance when retired
viii)   Goal setting to prepare for retirement.

---

can be achieved post-retirement (Mojon-Azzi et al., 2007). This supported the change in the session towards becoming a half-day workshop examining lifestyle and occupations. The content shown in Box 5.2 particularly concerns how retirement can bring about loss in terms of identity, routine, status and balance (Jonsson et al., 2000). The issue of retirement is of particular interest to occupational therapists and healthy ageing is particularly relevant (Pereira & Stagnitti, 2008). Again, by providing occupation-focussed interventions (which have been so popular that the session is now a permanent feature on this tri-monthly programme), illustrates the power and relevance of occupational therapy within workplace contexts.

Conclusion

Work-based well-being programmes are nothing new. Historically, they have been either bought in from private companies supplying stress and lifestyle management techniques or provided by in-house training teams. What is not so common is an occupational therapist providing a variety of techniques and strategies, despite being suitably trained and providing a holistic approach to individuals (Stein & Cutler, 2002). The possible contributions that occupational therapists can make to work-based well-being programmes have been presented. Working with well populations and taking on a health promotion role is not particularly innovative within the occupational therapy profession, however, few have applied these within worksites, nor have many UK-based occupational therapists stepped outside of traditional statutory health care to work alongside occupational health and human resources teams.

   This chapter demonstrates how an occupational therapist can contribute to staff well-being strategies at work. More significantly by working at corporate level and in collaboration with other professionals, it is possible to start to change the cultural context of the workplace. Time spent in productive roles and occupations can be the longest yet least satisfying, especially if the motivation for engaging in paid work is purely for fiscal reasons. There is some potential in supporting people at work to combat potential stressors, address life imbalance and increase quality leisure time. The profession of occupational therapy appears to have missed a trick here. Occupational therapists need to recognise and positively assert themselves within their own work bases. Taking an occupational perspective and their skills to their employer and offering to share these with others is one way to promote the effectiveness of the profession. By offering to work alongside occupational health teams within their organisations, a collaborative, multi-disciplinary approach can be achieved. Contributing well-being and lifestyle programmes that have been piloted on 'well' staff members could convince reluctant managers that development of skills in lifestyle and well-being can ultimately benefit the client. Conversely, occupational therapists who have developed skills which enhance occupational performance and therefore well-being (e.g. in fatigue, and stress management, and/or occupational balance) within the statutory organisations; could offer packages to private employers thus providing 'third stream' income to the statutory sector or as an enterprise initiative. Ultimately, by actively promoting the profession and capitalising on opportunities to contribute professional skills, occupational therapists can carve a path that is not only rewarding but makes in-roads into an avenue of future practice that could pay a dividend for personal and professional growth.

References

Anand-Keller, P., Lehmann, D., & Milligan, K. (2009). Effectiveness of corporate well-being programmes. *Journal of Macromarketing, 29* (3), 279–230

Argyle, M. (2001). *The Psychology of Happiness.* New York: Taylor & Francis.

Aromaa, A., & Koskinen, S. (2004). *Health and Functional Capacity in Finland: Baseline Results of the Health 2000 Health Examination Survey.* Helsinki: National Public Health Institute.

Aguiar, M., & Hurst, E. (2007). Measuring trends in leisure: The allocation of time over five decades. *Quarterly Journal of Economics, 122* (3), 969–1006.

Bertera, R. L. (1990). The effects of workplace health promotion on absenteeism and employment costs in a large industrial population. *American Journal of Public Health, 80* (9), 1101–1105.

Black, C. (2008). *Dame Carol Black's Review of the Health of Britain's Working Age Population Working for a Healthier Tomorrow.* London: TSO.

Booth, A. O., Nowson, C. A., Matters, & H. (2008). Evaluation of an interactive, tailored. Internet-based weight loss programme: A pilot study. *Health Education Research, 23,* 371–381.

Burke, R. (2009). Working to live or living to work: Should individuals and organizations care? *Journal of Business Ethics, 84* (1), 167–172.

Burns, T., Catty, J., White, S., Becker, T., Koletsi, M., Fioritti, A., Réossler, W., Tomov, T., van Busschbach, J., Wiersma, D., & Lauber, C. (2009). The Impact of Supported Employment and Working on Clinical and Social Functioning: Results of an International Study of Individual Placement and Support. *Schizophrenia Bulletin. 35* (5), 949–958.

Carroll, D., Smith, G. D., Shipley, M. J., Steptoe, A., Brunner, E. J., & Marmot, M. G. (2001). Blood pressure reactions to acute psychological stress and future blood pressure status: A 10-year follow-up of men in the Whitehall II Study. *Psychosomatic Medicine, 63* (5), 737–743.

Catty, J., Lissouba, P., White, S., Becker, T., Drake, R. E., Fioritti, A., Knapp, M., Lauber, C., Rossler, W., Tomov, T., van Busschbach, J., Wiersma, D., & Burns, T. (2008). Predictors of employment for people with severe mental illness: Results of an international six-centre randomised controlled trial. *The British Journal of Psychiatry: the Journal of Mental Science. 192* (3), 224–231.

Christiansen, C., & Townsend, E. (2004). The occupational nature of communities. In Christiansen, C., & Townsend, E. (Eds.), *Introduction to Occupation: The Art and Science of Living* (pp. 141–172). New Jersey: Prentice Hall.

Christiansen, C. H., & Matuska (2006) Lifestyle balance: A review of concepts and research. *Journal of Occupational Science, 13* (1), 49–61.

Chiuve, S. E, McCullough, M.L., Sacks, F.M, & Rimm, E. B. (2006). Healthy lifestyle factors in the primary prevention of coronary heart disease among men: Benefits among users and nonusers of lipid-lowering and antihypertensive medications. *Circulation, 114* (2), 160–167.

Clark, F., Azen, S, P., Zemke, R., Jackson, J., Calson, M., Mandel, D., Hay, J., Josephson, K., Cherry, B., Hessel, C., Jocelynne, P., & Lipson, L. (1997) Occupational therapy for independent-living older adults: A randomized controlled trial. *JAMA, 278* (16), 1321–1326

Chatzitheochari, S., & Arber, S. (2009). Lack of sleep, work and the long hours culture: evidence from the UK Time Use Survey. *Work, Employment and Society, 23* (1), 30–48.

Childress, J. M., & Lindsay, G. M. (2006). National indications of increasing investment in workplace health promotion programmes by large- and medium-size companies. *North Carolina Medical Journal, 67* (6), 449–452.

Clemson, L. (2009). Preventing Falls in the Elderly Using "Stepping On": A Group-Based Education Programme. *International Handbook of Occupational Therapy Interventions.* New York: Springer.

Clemson, L., Cusick, A., & Fozzard, C. (1999). Managing risk and exerting control: determining follow through with falls prevention. *Disability and Rehabilitation, 21* (12), 531–541.

Colton, C.W, & Manderscheid, R. W. (2006). Congruencies in increased mortality rates, years of potential life lost, and causes of death among public mental health clients in eight states. *Preventing Chronic Disease, 3* (2).

Craig, L. (2006). Does father care mean fathers share? A comparison of how mothers and fathers in intact families spend time with children. *Gender And Society, 20* (2), 259–281.

Cook, R. F., Billings, D. W., Hersch, R. K., Back, A. S, & Hendrickson, A. (2007). A field test of a web-based workplace health promotion programme to improve dietary practices, reduce stress, and increase physical activity: Randomized controlled trial. *Journal of Medical Internet Research, 9* (2).

Creed, P. A., & Macintyre, S. R. (2001) The relative effects of deprivation of the latent and manifest benefits of employment on the well-being of unemployed people. *Journal of Occupational Health Psychology, 6* (4), 324–331.

Creek, J., & Lougher, L. (2008). *Occupational Therapy and Mental Health.* Edinburgh: Churchill Livingstone Elsevier.

Curran, C., Knapp, M., McDaid, D., Támasson, K., & Group, T. M. (2007). Mental health and employment: An overview of patterns and policies across Western Europe. *Journal of Mental Health, 16* (2), 195–209.

Dantzer, C., Wardle, J., Fuller, R., Pampalone, S. Z., & Steptoe, A., (2006). International Study of Heavy Drinking: Attitudes and Socio-demographic Factors in University Students. *Journal of American College Health, 55* (2), 83–90.

Dave, D., Rashad, I., & Spasojevic, J. (2006). *The Effects of Retirement on Physical and Mental Health Outcomes.* Cambridge, MA: National Bureau of Economic Research.

Department for Work and Pensions. (2002). *Pathways to Work: Helping People into Employment.* London: HMSO.

Department of Health (DoH). (2004). *Choosing Health: Making Healthy Choices Easier.* London: HMSO.

Department of Health (DoH). (2006) *The Health Act 2006: Code of Practice for the Prevention and Control of Healthcare Associated Infections.* London: HMSO.

Diener, E., Oishi, S., & Lucas, R. E. (2003). PERSONALITY PROCESSES - Personality, culture, and subjective well-being: Emotional and cognitive evaluations of life. *Annual Review of Psychology, 54,* 403–426.

Eid, M., & Larsen, R. J. (2008). *The Science of Subjective Well-Being.* New York: Guilford Press.

Faragher, E. B., Cass, M., & Cooper, C. L, (2005). The relationship between job satisfaction and health: A meta-analysis. *Occupational and Environmental Medicine, 62* (2), 105–112.

Gerdtham, U. G., & Johannesson, M., (2003). A note on the effect of unemployment on mortality. *Journal of Health Economics, 22*: 505–518.

Goetzel, R. Z., Long, S. R., Ozminkowski, R. J., Hawkins, K., Wang, S., & Lynch, W. (2004). Health, absence, disability, and presenteeism cost estimates of certain physical and mental health conditions affecting U.S. Employers. *Journal of Occupational and Environmental Medicine, 46* (4): 398–412.

Goetzel, R. Z, & Ozminkowski, R. J. (2008). The health and cost benefits of work site health-promotion programmes. *Annual Review of Public Health. 29,* 303–23.

Goetzel, R. Z., Ozminkowski, R. J., Bruno, J. A., Rutter, K. R., Isaac, F, & Wang, S. (2002). The long-term impact of Johnson & Johnson's Health & Wellness Programme on employee health risks. *Journal of Occupational and Environmental Medicine/American College of Occupational and Environmental Medicine, 44* (5), 417–424.

Grawitch, M. J., Trares, S., & Kohler, J. M. (2007). Healthy workplace practices and employee outcomes. *International Journal Of Stress Management, 14* (3), 275–293.

Griffiths, K., & Christensen, H. (2006). Review of randomised controlled trials of Internet interventions for mental disorders and related conditions. *Clinical Psychologist, 10* (1), 16–29.

Groenvold, M., Petersen, M., Idler, E., Bjorner, J., Fayers, P., & Mouridsen, H. (2007). Psychological distress and fatigue predicted recurrence and survival in primary breast cancer patients. *Breast Cancer Research and Treatment, 105* (2), 209–219.

Grzywacz, J. G., & Marks, N.F. (2000). Reconceptualising the work-family interface: An Ecological perspective on the correlates of positive and negative spillover between work and family. *Journal of Occupational Health Psychology, 5,* 111–126.

Hagedorn, R. (2000). *Tools for Practice in Occupational Therapy: A Structured Approach to Core Skills and Processes.* Edinburgh: Churchill Livingstone.

Hagedorn, R. (2001). *Foundations for Practice in Occupational Therapy.* Edinburgh: Churchill Livingstone.

Hammell, K. W. (2004). Using qualitative evidence to inform theories of occupation. In: K. W. Hammell, & C. Carpenter (Eds.), *Qualitative Research in Evidence-Based Rehabilitation* (pp. 14–26). Edinburgh: Churchill Livingstone.

Health and Safety Executive: Great Britain. (2003). *Real Solutions, Real People: A Manager's Guide to Tackling Work-Related Stress.* Norwich: HSE.

Health and Safety Executive: Great Britain. (2005). *Working Together to Reduce Stress at Work: A Guide for Employees. England.* Norwich: HSE.

Health and Safety Executive. (2007). *Managing the Causes of Work-Related Stress: A Step-by-Step Approach to Using the Management Standards.* Norwich: HSE.

Henderson, M., Glozier, N., & Elliott, K. H. (2005). Editorials – Long term sickness absence. *British Medical Journal, 330* (7495), 802

Holmes, J. (2007). *Vocational Rehabilitation.* Oxford: Blackwell Publishing.

Houston, D., Meyer, L. H., & Paewai, S. (2006) Academic staff workloads and job satisfaction: expectations and values in academe, *Journal of Higher Education Policy and Management, 28* (1), 17–30.

Hughes, R (2008). Older people falling out of bed; risk restraint. *The British Journal of Occupational Therapy, 71* (9), 389–392.

Jonsson, H., Borell, L., & Sadlo, G. (2000). Retirement: An occupational transition with consequences for temporality, balance and meaning of occupations. *Journal of Occupational Science, 7* (1), 29–37.

Kielhofner, G. (2002) *A Model of Human Occupation: Theory and Application* (4th ed.). Philadelphia: Lippincott Williams & Wilkins.

Kinman, G. (2008). Work stressors, health and sense of coherence in UK academic employees. *Educational Psychology. 28* (7), 823–835.

Kreis, J., & Bödeker, W. (2004). *Health-related and economic benefits of workplace health promotion and prevention: Summary of the scientific evidence*. Essen: BKK Bundesverband. http://www.enwhp.org/download/IGA-Report_3_English.pdf.

Kumar, R., & Kumar, S. (2008). Musculoskeletal risk factors in cleaning occupation – A literature review. *International Journal of Industrial Ergonomics, 38* (2), 158.

Kurth, T., Moore, S. C., Gaziano, M. J., Kase, C. S., Stampfer, M. J.; Berger, K., & Buring, J. E. (2006). Healthy lifestyle and the risk of stroke in women. *Arch Intern Med, 166* (13): 1403–1409.

Law, M., & Baum, C. (2005). Measurement in occupational therapy In C. Christiansen, C. M. Baum, & J. Bass-Haugen (Eds.), *Occupational Therapy Performance, Participation, and Well-Being*. Thorofare, NJ: Slack.

Layard, R. (2005). *Happiness: Lessons from a New Science*. London: Allen Lane.

Linnan, L., Bowling, M., Childress, J., Lindsay, G., Blakey, C., Royall, P., Pronk, S., Wieker, S. (2008). Results of the 2004 National Worksite Health Promotion Survey. *American Journal of Public Health, 98* (8), 1503–1509.

Matuska, K. M., & Christiansen, C. (2009). *Life Balance: Multidisciplinary Theories and Research*. Thorofare, NJ: SLACK.

McKenna, J., & Thew, M. (2008) Getting the balance right: Managing work-home conflict. In M. Thew & J. McKenna (Eds.), *Lifestyle Management in Health and Social Care*. Oxford: Blackwell/Wiley Publishing.

Mellor, G., & St John, W. (2007). Occupational health nurses' perceptions of their current and future roles. *Journal of Advanced Nursing, 58* (6), 585–593.

Mojon-Azzi, S., Sousa-Poza, A., & Widmer, R. (2007). The effect of retirement on health: a panel analysis using data from the Swiss Household Panel. *Swiss Medical Weekly : Official Journal of the Swiss Society of Infectious Diseases, the Swiss Society of Internal Medicine, the Swiss Society of Pneumology, 137*, 41–42.

Mountain, G., Mozley, C., Craigl, C., & Ball, L. (2008). Occupational therapy led health promotion for older people: Feasibility of the lifestyle matters programme. *The British Journal of Occupational Therapy, 71* (10), 406.

National Institute for Clinical Excellence (NICE). (2004). *Anxiety: Management of Anxiety (Panic Disorder, with or without Agoraphobia, and Generalised Anxiety Disorder) Adults in Primary, Secondary and Community Care*. (Clinical guideline 22). London: NICE.

Neville L. M., O'Hara B., & Milat A. J. (2009). Computer-tailored dietary behaviour change interventions: A systematic review. *Health Education Research, 24* (4), 699–720.

Oakley, K. (2002). *Occupational Health Nursing*. London: Whurr.

Pelletier, K. R. (2005). A review and analysis of the clinical and cost-effectiveness studies of comprehensive health promotion and disease management programmes at the worksite: Update VI 2000–2004. *Journal of Occupational and Environmental Medicine, 47* (10): 1051–1058.

Pelletier, B., Boles, M., & Lynch, W. (2004). Change in health risks and work productivity over time. *Journal of Occupational and Environmental Medicine, 46* (7),746–754.

Pereira, R., & Stagnitti, K. (2008). The meaning of leisure for well-elderly Italians in an Australian community: Implications for occupational therapy. *Australian Occupational Therapy Journal, 55*, 39–46.

Rahtz, D., & Szykman, L. (2008). Can health care organizations better contribute to quality of life by focusing on preventive health knowledge? *Journal of Macromarketing, 28* (2), 122–129.

Ross, J. (2007). *Occupational Therapy and Vocational Rehabilitation*. Chichester, England: John Wiley and Sons.

Roulstone, A. (2003). *Thriving and Surviving at Work: Disabled People's Employment Strategies*. Bristol, UK: Policy Press.

Ryan, R. M., & Deci, E. L. (2001). On happiness and human potentials: A review of research on hedonic and eudaimonic well-being. *Annual Review of Psychology, 52*, 141–166.

Salmi, P., Svedberg, P., Hagberg, J., Lundh, G., Linder, J., & Alexanderson, K. (2009). Outcome of multidisciplinary investigations of long-term sickness absentees. *Disability & Rehabilitation, 31* (2), 131–137.

Siahpush, M., Spittal, M., & Singh, G. K. (2008). Happiness and life satisfaction prospectively predict self-rated health, physical health, and the presence of limiting, long-term health conditions. *American Journal of Health Promotion : AJHP, 23* (1) 18–26.

Simpson, J., Oldenburg, B., Owen, N., Harris, D., Dobbins, T., & Salmon, A. (2000). The Australian national workplace health project: Design and baseline findings. *Preventative Medicine, 31*, 249–260.

Stein, F., & Cutler, S. K. (2002). *Psychosocial Occupational Therapy: A Holistic Approach*. Australia: Delmar/Thomson Learning.

Thew, M. (2008a). Portable relaxation. In M. Thew & J. McKenna (Eds) (2008) *Lifestyle Management in Health and Social Care*. Oxford: Blackwell/ Wiley Publishing.

Thew, M. (2008b). Sleep- The life Enhancer. In M. Thew & J. McKenna (Eds) (2008) *Lifestyle Management in Health and Social Care*. Oxford: Blackwell/Wiley Publishing.

Thew, M., & McKenna, J. (2008). *Lifestyle Management in Health and Social Care*. Oxford: Blackwell Publishing.

Thew, M., & Pemberton, S. (2008) Energy for life. In M. Thew & J. McKenna (Eds.), *Lifestyle Management in Health and Social Care*. Oxford: Blackwell/Wiley Publishing.

Tsai, S. P., Wendt, J. K., Donnelly, R. P., Jong, G. D., & Ahmed, F. S. (2005). Age at retirement and long term survival of an industrial population: Prospective cohort study. *BMJ : British Medical Journal, 331* (7523), 995.

Tytherleigh, M. Y., Webb, C., Cooper, C. L., & Ricketts, C. (2005). Occupational stress in UK higher education institutions: A comparative study of all staff categories. *Higher Education Research and Development, 24* (1), 41–61.

van Straten, A., Cuijpers, P., & Smits, N. (2008). Effectiveness of a web-based self-help intervention for symptoms of depression, anxiety, and stress: Randomized controlled trial. *Journal of Medical Internet Research, 10* (1), e7.

Velde, B., & Fidler, G. (2002). *Lifestyle Performance: A Model for Engaging in the Power of Occupation*. Thorofare, NJ: Slack.

de Vries G., & Schene, A. H. (2009). Reintegration into work of people suffering from depression. In I. Söderback (Ed.), *International Handbook of Occupational Therapy Interventions*. Dordrecht: Springer.

Waddell, G, Burton, A. (2006) *Is Work Good for Your Health and Well Being*? London: TSO.

Wanless, D. (2004). *Securing Good Health for the Whole Population: Final Report*. Norwich: H.M.S.O.

Whiteford, G., Klomp, N, & Wright St-Clair, V. (2005). In G. Whiteford, & Clair V. W.-S. (Eds.), *Occupation & Practice in Context* (pp. 3–15). Marickville, NSW: Elsevier Churchill Livingstone.

Wilcock, A. A. (1998). *An Occupational Perspective of Health*. Thorofare: SLACK.

Wilcock, A. A. (2005). Occupational science: Bridging occupation and health. *Canadian Journal of Occupational Therapy. Revue Canadienne D'ergothérapie. 72* (1), 5–12.

Wilcock, A. A. (2006). *An Occupational Perspective of Health*. Thorofare, NJ: SLACK.

World Health Organization (WHO). (1995). *Global Strategy on Occupational Health for All: The Way to Health at Work*. Geneva: WHO.

World Health Organization (WHO). (2001). *The Role of the Occupational Health Nurse in Workplace Health Management*. Copenhagen: WHO Regional Office for Europe.

World Health Organization (WHO). (2002). *The World Health Report: Reducing Risks, Promoting Healthy Life*. Geneva: WHO.

World Health Organization (WHO). (2005). *Mental Health Policies and Programmes in the Workplace*. Geneva: WHO.

Zuzanek, J., (1998) Time use, time pressure, personal stress, mental health and life satisfaction from a life cycle perspective. *Journal of Occupational Science*, 5 (1), 26–39.

Chapter 6

An occupational perspective of a disability-focused employment service

Sally Hall

Work saves us from the three great evils of life: boredom, vice and need.

(Voltaire, 1759)

Introduction

Well-being and health are closely associated with feeling productive and worthwhile, as has been argued in previous chapters. This chapter focuses more closely on the role that occupational therapists can play in supporting people who have disabilities or chronic health conditions or problems to be and feel more productive particularly through paid employment. Productivity is a key tenet of occupational therapy models such as the Canadian Model of Occupational Performance (Law et al., 1996). It has been defined as "a contribution to the social and economic fabric of the community" (Townsend, 2002, p. 34) and is understood to refer to occupations undertaken throughout the lifespan, from a child's schoolwork to the employment, home maintenance and parenting occupations of adulthood (Ross, 2007). This definition of productivity encompasses a much wider range of occupations than simply paid employment or 'work'. However, work lies at the heart of our society's collective understanding of what it is to be productive – and is one of the most important means by which we make a positive contribution to our communities, our families and our own personal development.

Despite the arguments and evidence that connect occupational therapy with work related issues, it is clear that such opportunities are not widely available within the usual range of placements on offer to student occupational therapists. It is indicative of the current trend within occupational therapy practice within the UK to work within a medical or specialist condition focussed paradigm and not a vocational one, leaving many occupational therapists with little or no experience of applying their skills in facilitating returning people to paid work (COT, 2007). Therefore, a role emerging placement setting provided the most apposite opportunity to gain valuable skills and to explore the potential contribution of an occupational perspective within an existing vocational rehabilitation setting. The College of Occupational Therapists advises occupational therapy students to actively seek placements which reflect the rising flexibility in workplace patterns, in order

Role Emerging Occupational Therapy: Maximising Occupation-Focused Practice, 1st edition. Edited by Miranda Thew, Mary Edwards, Sue Baptiste and Matthew Molineux. © 2011 Blackwell Publishing Ltd.

to open up opportunities for innovative practice (COT, 2004, p. 21). Such placements offer the opportunity to critically evaluate an existing service and to prompt reflection on the possible development of more occupationally focused services in future. With this mandate in mind, a role emerging placement was located in a welfare-to-work-focused employment service. This chapter offers an exploration and reflection of a role emerging placement which demonstrates the development of skills and knowledge in addressing work-related issues, and offers tangible examples of innovative possibilities for future occupational therapy practice in this area.

A need to be productive

The need to feel and be productive can be illustrated with an account of one woman's experience, as heard by the author; a narrative which was delivered with great courage by the woman herself speaking at a conference for health professionals. Taking to the stage, she openly talked of her recent suicide attempt following a violent relationship which had eroded her self-esteem and left her severely depressed. Told she was 'useless' more often than she could remember, she had long ago begun to believe it. She felt dissociated from society and dislocated from her support networks. But after engaging with the local mental health services, she was offered an opportunity to engage in a programme of vocational rehabilitation provided by a local charity. She started with voluntary work in a field she found meaningful, and gradually, her confidence began to return as she worked towards increasing both time commitments and task complexity. Attending a series of job-skills-focused workshops, she was then supported through the process of applying for paid employment. Now working full-time, her resilience had been strengthened to such an extent that she even felt able to discuss her experiences in public.

This woman's profoundly moving narrative demonstrated a 'real world' application of the theoretical view that work can be both a vehicle for healing and a means of enabling occupational justice (Jakobsen, 2004). In 2006, a robust and extensive systematic review found that work met important psychosocial needs, and was central to individual identity, social roles and social status in societies where employment was the cultural norm. Conversely, lack of paid employment was associated with higher mortality, and poorer physical and mental health (Waddell & Burton, 2006). This evidence was cited in the influential Black review, 'Working for a Healthier Tomorrow' (Black, 2008), and is further mirrored by occupational therapy literature, which has demonstrated that work enables individuals to structure time and routines, make social connections and achieve both self-efficacy and a sense of purpose (Kennedy-Jones et al., 2005; Lloyd & Waghorn, 2007; Ross, 2007). Furthermore, income generated by paid employment enables the pursuit of valued leisure occupations and provides a means of meeting health and social needs (Jakobsen, 2004). As the College of Occupational Therapists (COT) states: "To work in paid employment is to become part of our society: to be included rather than excluded." (COT, 2007, p. 2).

The service

The role emerging placement was with a disability-focused employment service which had formerly provided primarily factory-based employment for people with disabilities across the UK. In recent years the business model for this service had been reformulated, resulting in the closure of many of the factories. Instead, a national network of high-street branches had been established, with the aim of enabling people with a range of disabilities and health conditions (such as neurological and musculoskeletal conditions, learning disabilities, and mental health problems such as depression and schizophrenia) access mainstream employment opportunities. In 2008, the service had a national target of helping 20,000 people a year to access paid work by 2012. A 'job entry' involving a minimum of 16 hours per week of paid employment was the primary measure of success. The service motto was 'putting ability first'. This reflected the conclusions of the Black review, which called for the introduction of the 'fit-note' to enable people with health conditions to focus on their strengths and abilities rather than limitations (Black, 2008, p. 12). It also implicitly accords with an occupational perspective, which avoids a narrow biomedical focus on impairment and aims to engage with the individual (Turner, 2002; Finlay, 2004), and harnessing clients' abilities (and interests) to facilitate engagement in meaningful occupation (Blesedell Crepeau et al., 2003).

Individuals using the service were referred to as 'candidates'; the service was limited to serving candidates, aged between 16–65, who received certain benefits, or who were recent education-leavers. Candidates whose benefits were not disability related were eligible for the service if they had a diagnosed disability or health condition. Referrals usually came through from the local government-funded employment agency and social security office and local colleges, but occasionally also through health professionals, including an occupational therapist working with young men who had experienced traumatic brain injury. Individual self-referrals were also accepted but were rare in practice.

City-wide referrals were received and processed at the local branch office, which was located in the city centre. None of the staff (known as employment advisors) involved in the process at the time of the role emerging placement had a background or qualification as a health professional. Most had been recruited from mainstream recruitment or specialist employment agencies, and all staff had some voluntary experience in health or social care, with community-based voluntary work actively encouraged. In addition to the employment advisors, members of the team included two liaison officers working in partnership with colleges and local employers, and a retention specialist who continued to work with candidates for up to one year post-employment.

Following a referral, an initial interview focusing on the candidate's skills, interests and previous employment history was carried out. At this stage, candidates were also asked briefly about the impact of their disability. Following this initial interview, the employment advisor determined whether to refer the candidate to one of two areas of support:

i) The Recruitment arm of the service involved candidates attending regular 'Job Action Groups', where the employment advisors assisted them to match their skills and abilities to existing vacancies, and provided support with the job application process.
ii) The Development candidates participated in a 'Key Skills programme', which involved attending motivational workshops, sessions on curriculum vitae (CV) writing, mock job interviews and visits to likely employers.

There was an expectation that Development candidates would progress to become a Recruitment candidate shortly after completing this programme. However, some required extra support, such as budgeting assistance, work task modification and graded exposure to public transport. The implementation of such support necessitated an implicitly occupational focus. For example, the role involved conducting activity analysis of job tasks to enable modifications to the occupation, the person or the environment. Occupations such as using public transport were graded or adapted to fit the individual's capabilities. One member of staff was employed specifically to offer this extra support. Although the skills, perspectives and strategies of this role appeared to arise innately from an occupational perspective, there was no expectation that it would be performed by a qualified occupational therapist.

Socio-political context of the service

The lack of health professional input in this service reflected the national trend over the past five years towards the provision of vocational rehabilitation primarily by the Department for Work and Pensions-funded rather than Department of Health-funded UK agencies. Defined as: "A process by which those disadvantaged by illness or disability can be enabled to access, return to, or remain in employment, or other useful occupation" (British Society of Rehabilitation Medicine, 2003), vocational rehabilitation was once routinely offered by health professionals in both physical rehabilitation and mental health settings, usually within occupational therapy departments (Holmes, 2007; Ross, 2007). However, as the National Health Service has increasingly focused on acute care (Grahame, 2002; Joss, 2002; Alsop, 2004; Robdale, 2004; Holmes, 2007), opportunities to deliver vocational rehabilitation in health care settings have significantly diminished. Indeed, many occupational therapists in the UK now have "little or no experience of applying their skills to work-related issues, or of becoming involved with workplace rehabilitation" (COT, 2007, p. 1).

Contextualised by a socio-political framework that separates 'work' from 'health', vocational rehabilitation is now offered primarily from a 'welfare-to-work' perspective, particularly to those who are already in receipt of disability benefits. This contrasts with the systematic implementation of vocational rehabilitation within the health service in countries such as the Netherlands, where inpatients are routinely offered 'employment reintegration' programmes (Schonherr et al, 2004). In Germany, Austria, Sweden and Spain, a request for benefits due to accident or illness automatically generates a referral to health services for vocational rehabilitation (Frank & Sawney, 2003). The locus of control for provision of services therefore resides primarily within the health service, differing significantly from the UK model.

It is worth considering the cultural, political and institutional context when reflecting on the significance of this role emerging placement. On a practical level, there is now scant opportunity in traditional clinical settings for occupational therapy students to develop nascent skills in vocational rehabilitation (Holmes, 2007, p. 4). Yet the occupational therapy profession is unlikely to regain a place in the provision of vocational rehabilitation services without the development of appropriate placements through which students may develop vocationally focused skills and knowledge. This highlights the value of such a placement in developing new areas of practice for the profession and ensuring occupational therapy is influential in key areas such as vocational rehabilitation with which there is such a natural, and historically grounded, fit.

Applying an occupational perspective

The benchmark strategy for implementing vocational rehabilitation programmes in England and Wales was outlined by the Government in a 2002 Green Paper, Pathways to Work (DWP, 2002), which set a target of facilitating paid employment for one million claimants of Incapacity Benefit by 2015 (DWP, 2008). Through this strategy, specialist employment agencies were tasked with removing barriers to work for benefits claimants (Blyth, 2006). The Welfare Reform Act (2007) further reinforced this approach, instituting mandatory engagement with a work-focused programme for those claiming the new Employment and Support Allowance (ESA). In many ways, this approach chimes implicitly with an occupational perspective, which considers the relationship between a person, their occupations and their environment (Law et al., 1996), and recognises that environmental barriers such as lack of access to transport or social stigma may impact on employment status to an even greater extent than the individual's disability or health condition (Riddell, 2002; Mercer, 2005). Yet the current focus on removing barriers to work reflects only one aspect of an occupational perspective which, if implemented more holistically, could provide the locus for more a person-centred service provision.

Despite the erosion of professional influence that has been experienced in the area (Holmes, 2007; Ross, 2007), occupational therapists are still widely considered to be the most appropriate professionals to deliver vocational rehabilitation (Joss, 2002, 2007; Royal College of Psychiatrists, 2002; Alsop, 2004; Kennedy-Jones et al, 2005; Holmes, 2007; Ross, 2007; Thurgood & Frank, 2007). This is predominantly because the profession offers expertise in activity analysis, the grading and adaptation of occupations, and the matching of functional capabilities to the demands of a task. But an occupational perspective also runs deeper. Its focus is on the person, in addition to the environment and the occupation. This necessitates an understanding of the impact of ill-health on the individual's ability to perform occupations. It demands the ability to provide interventions that focus on individual well-being as well as external job entry targets. It requires an understanding of productivity that is not purely limited to paid employment. Most importantly of all, it is based on the holistic understanding that a person's spirituality (Law et al., 1996) or volition (Kielhofner, 2002) is key to achieving sustainable positive outcomes. As Holmes states: "Modern vocational rehabilitation should not be about trying to fit people into pigeonholes of services just to meet the outcome requirements of funding. Motivational issues should be [at the heart] of the programme" (Holmes, 2007, p. 13).

Initiating change

The primary objective of this role emerging placement was to develop a sustainable, realistic and measurable project which could be implemented within a six-week period, and which would demonstrate an occupational perspective. In attempting to apply such a perspective to this service, it was necessary to reflect on the limitations of what might be possible. Nationally, the service was tasked with specific and ambitious targets. It was apparent that any project which appeared to divert from these targets would not achieve sustainable success that could be measured in a meaningful way for the service needs.

In considering appropriate directions for the project, reflection initially focused on means of harnessing candidates' individual interests and motivations to achieve more sustainable job entry outcomes. However, such ideas did not appear to complement the service aims. Candidates may have aspired to engage in productive occupations that were meaningful to them as individuals, but the focus of the service was in accessing available (mainly paid) job opportunities rather than creating individually tailored work pathways. Given the job entry targets that guided service provision, it was in some ways counterproductive to encourage a candidate to develop interests and skills in an area where they would be unlikely to find employment within a short space of time. This factor emerged through detailed discussion with the service manager and other members of the team. Such a consultation process was an essential aspect of developing the project. Each member of the team offered a different perspective, and it became apparent that some were more open to suggestions for developing the service than others. Following the strategies advocated by Brent Braveman to enable effective management of change within occupational therapy (Braveman 2006, pp.197–214), a key change agent was identified and his opinion sought prior to rolling out ideas more widely to the team. As advocated by Braveman, the change agent was both open to new ideas and skilled in supporting the implementation of ideas in practice (Braveman, 2006, p. 202).

In general, the team reflected a general societal trend in that most were not conversant with the philosophy and practice of occupational therapy. In order to offer a clear understanding of the objectives of the placement and why a student occupational therapist had been placed there, a presentation titled 'What Is an Occupational Perspective?' was delivered to the team. Again, this was informed by Braveman's work on communication strategies for effectively managing change, which advises holding carefully planned communication events involving all team members, with time for questions and answers (Braveman, 2006, p. 208). The presentation provided an opportunity to demonstrate synergies between a occupational perspective and the ability-focused service philosophy, as well as provided a forum to solicit suggestions and observe levels of interest. It prompted a useful discussion, particularly around the issues of motivation in seeking paid employment.

Eventually, through observation, discussion and reflection, it became apparent that there was a gap in the service which could potentially benefit immediately from an occupationally focused approach. Employment advisors were not health professionals, therefore they were not focusing on the impact of unmet health needs on occupational performance. The service motto of putting ability first also appeared to provide a frame of reference which discouraged an emphasis on the impact of health conditions or disabilities. As a result, candidates were moving forward through the recruitment process with little support or attention paid to issues such as pain, low mood and anxiety which had the potential to directly affect their employability. For example, a candidate in receipt of benefits due to chronic back pain may have gone on to develop low mood or anxiety after several months of unemployment. Although this may not have been picked up by a GP or other health professionals, it could potentially have a direct impact on the process of applying for and undertaking paid employment. It was therefore decided that the aim of the project would be to ascertain levels of unmet health needs such as this, and to develop a pathway to enable such needs to be better met.

Throughout this reflection process, support was offered by a senior occupational therapist who acted as an off-site practice placement educator. Weekly supervision provided a forum for careful consideration of team dynamics, enabling creative thinking about how to encourage a shift in practice within the team as a whole to consider health and social issues.

The project

Although the emphasis on ability rather than disability was certainly a positive aspect of this service, there were limitations to this model of practice. With no health professionals involved in vocational rehabilitation processes, there was little consideration for the ongoing impact of health conditions on occupational performance. Consequently, it appeared that a large proportion of candidates were attempting to gain employment with unmet health needs which were then directly impacting on their everyday function, and therefore their success in gaining employment. It was considered necessary to devise an assessment tool to determine the impact of unmet health needs on levels of occupational performance. This was intended to achieve several objectives:

  i) To provide an evidence base by quantifying the impact of candidates' unmet health needs on their ability to carry out daily occupations.
 ii) To highlight at an early stage any health issues affecting an individual candidate which may later prove to be a significant barrier to employment.
iii) To provide an opportunity to signpost candidates to specialist services in order to tackle these health issues.
iv) To support and enhance existing information pertaining to individuals in order to determine an appropriate match between candidates and vacancies.

Consequently, the 'General Health Profile' assessment tool was designed and developed (e.g. Figure x). The tool was function focused, with candidates asked if they 'struggled to do what they needed or wanted to do on a daily basis' as a result of commonly experienced symptoms in six key areas: pain, mobility issues, fatigue, insomnia, depression and anxiety. For example, candidates were asked if they had experienced 'feeling really tired' (fatigue), 'pain at night' (pain), 'feeling really bad about myself' (depression), 'stiff joints' (mobility), 'feeling on edge' (anxiety) or 'waking up really early' (insomnia) in the previous week. A rating scale ranging from 'none of the time' to 'all of the time' was provided for each of the 24 listed items. Candidates were also asked if they would be interested in further information or support with these issues. A total of 20 candidates completed this assessment tool. Strikingly, 90% experienced symptoms that prevented them doing everyday things at least some of the time; of those, 60% experienced anxiety, 40% sleep problems and 40% fatigue. Overall, 75% expressed an interest in further information or support.

It was recognised that candidates were likely to require a spectrum of support to address these unmet health needs. Therefore, a resource file named 'Highway to Health' was established. This file included an A–Z directory of local services to which candidates could be signposted, such as pain clinics, expert patient programmes and self-help workshops for those experiencing anxiety. In addition, a range of self-help material on subjects such as sleep, anxiety and anger management was collated and stored in the resource file to be distributed as appropriate. Finally, a number of flowcharts were devised to assist the service's employment advisors with interpreting the assessment tool and sourcing appropriate support. Another presentation was then given using hypothetical case studies to illustrate the process. For example, a candidate with chronic back pain experiencing further functional impairments as a result of low mood or anxiety might be signposted to primary care-based anxiety management clinics or community-based self-help programmes focusing on low mood. A candidate with significant pain might be referred to a pain clinic. If a client was experiencing mobility problems and may benefit from adaptations or equipment, links could be made to occupational therapists within the National Health Service to offer advice and support.

The experience

This role emerging placement gave rise to the development of a number of valuable skills. In general, the placement afforded a means of implementing change management strategies to create an achievable, sustainable outcome within a short period of time. Ideas for change were carefully considered and framed in accordance with key service targets: a crucial lesson for future practice. In terms of specific skills, knowledge of employment procedures was gained which would have been very difficult to replicate in a more traditional occupational therapy setting. Furthermore, the Highway to Health project was framed around a quantifiable evidence base, thereby encouraging and enabling the application of evidence-based practice. However, the most valuable aspect of the experience was the opportunity it provided to critically reflect on the current provision of 'welfare to work'-style vocational rehabilitation. It has already been argued that removing the health professionals' perspective from the process of vocational rehabilitation may result in a lack of recognition for the impact of unmet health needs on occupational performance: an observation which formed the basis of the Highway to Health project. Yet this project represented only one aspect of an occupational perspective. If an occupational therapist became involved in this service on a long-term basis, it would be hoped that there would be further opportunities to address the issues of motivation and to highlight the need for occupation to be meaningful in order to achieve sustainable targets. However, this objective may prove extremely challenging to implement within the constraints of the current welfare-to-work construct.

Due to its target-based funding structure, the service focused primarily on enabling people to transition from claiming benefits to undertaking paid employment. As a result, disabled people who were not eligible for benefits were not usually able to access the service, despite the fact that individuals attempting to retain employment have been widely identified as particularly likely to benefit from vocational rehabilitation (Joss,

2002; Robdale, 2004; Lloyd & Waghorn, 2007). Nationally, the service had begun to offer an additional package of support to employers keen to retain disabled employees, but this was provided on a consultancy basis, to be paid for by employers themselves, rather than as part of its publicly funded core service. There was no publicly funded support for those who were still on sick leave from work, for example, despite the call for early intervention made in the Black report (Black, 2008). The emphasis on paid employment also largely precluded education, voluntary work or part-time work of up to 16 hours per week from being identified as a successful outcome. Thus, there was little scope to assist candidates who wished to develop a new career or retrain completely. There was also little opportunity to work towards a graded entry into paid employment, for example, starting with voluntary work or part-time hours and increasing exposure over a period of time. With ambitious job entry targets to fulfil, the emphasis of this service was on high-volume vacancies in retail or domiciliary positions; work generally associated with minimum wage and low status. Whilst this may indeed have been the preferred area of work for many candidates, the complex relationship that links poverty, disability and lack of education (Roulstone & Barnes, 2005) remains unchallenged by this process. Paid employment can reinforce, rather than transcend, socio-economic divisions (Roulstone & Barnes, 2005), an observation which is particularly salient given that Incapacity Benefit claimants have been shown to be twice as likely as the general population to have no academic or vocational qualifications (Department of Work and Pensions, 2008).

Although the service provided was positive in many ways, and transformed the lives of hundreds of people, it was fundamentally limited by its obligations to fulfil the expectations of a welfare-to-work programme rather than the individual goals of the candidates themselves. The opportunity to implement a sustainable project was a valuable learning experience, but the real value of this role emerging placement was the chance it afforded to reflect on and seek out opportunities to practise with a more occupational focus, and to consider how a service might operate if framed by the wider definition of productivity identified by occupational therapy models.

The future: vocational rehabilitation

The occupational therapy profession has a crucial role to play in devising vocational rehabilitation services. However, opportunities for occupational therapists to practice vocational rehabilitation within the health service have eroded since the early 1990s, as work-focused interventions have come to be viewed as "superfluous to the business of an acute hospital" (Holmes, 2007, p. 4). As a consequence, facilitating a return to paid employment or possibly other productive occupations is rarely on the agenda. A system has therefore emerged whereby vocational rehabilitation is predominantly provided by services with a specific welfare-to-work mandate (Holmes, 2007, Ross, 2007).

It is widely believed that vocational rehabilitation is more likely to be successful if it takes place within a partnership model that integrates health care and employment services (Joss, 2002; Alsop, 2004; Bisiker & Millinchip, 2007; Holmes, 2007; Lloyd & Waghorn, 2007; Ross, 2007; Thurgood & Frank, 2007). This is the model which informs the Condition Management Programmes currently offered as part of the employment support component of the Pathways to Work strategy (Ross, 2007). However, such a partnership model could also move beyond the welfare-to-work paradigm to form the basis of an even more pioneering approach. This may involve developing organisations modelled on voluntary sector projects such as the 'Sunlight Trust', a community centre in Gillingham, Kent, which incorporates a high-street-style Fairtrade cafe run as a social enterprise by people with disabilities, health conditions or other barriers to employment. In 2008, the Trust supported 70 people to gain catering qualifications, while offering valuable opportunities to develop work-based skills (The Sunlight Trust, 2010). In addition, Sunlight operates a community-based radio station, a market garden, a childcare facility and a recording studio. All initiatives within the trust are social enterprises, therefore providing a business-focused experience for participants engaging in 'real world' occupations. Crucially, the project is actively based on a community partnership model, with enterprises managed collaboratively between 'service users' and 'staff'.

An occupational therapy-led initiative could model much of what is provided by Sunlight, while also incorporating the graded approach of the Australian clubhouse model cited by Kennedy-Jones et al (2005). This may involve a more formalised progression from voluntary roles within the project itself to managed work placements in the wider community, and eventually into open employment. Furthermore, the initiative would benefit from an explicitly client-centred focus, possibly utilising self-rated occupational therapy assessment tools, such as the Canadian Occupational Performance Measure (Law et al., 1996), to identify priority areas. A flexible approach to accommodating individual work goals could then be absorbed by the project, which would afford a varied range of opportunities determined by participants as well as managers. Such opportunities would fulfil a definition of productivity that includes, and also extends beyond, paid employment. Referrals could be accepted from health professionals in both primary and acute care, the charity sector, employment services or individuals themselves. Such an initiative could therefore provide a 'missing link' between the current provision offered by health care and employment services.

According to Ross (2007), occupational therapists need to consider how to expand their understanding of human occupation to arrive at an occupation-focused perspective of work. In addition to envisioning innovative services such as the project suggested above, this may also involve incremental changes within the existing system. Nominating a 'work champion' within each community mental health team has been identified as good practice (Ross, 2007). Further role emerging opportunities could also include placements in human resources departments of large employers, such as the National Health Service or local government, following a remit to focus on return-to-work practices, implementation of diversity strategies and guidance on reasonable adjustments, as defined by the Disability Discrimination Act 2005. Finally, a simple commitment to asking 'the work question' within health care environments – and 'the health question' within disability-focused employment services – may initiate the forging of links between the two paradigms

The future: personal practice

The true value of a role emerging placement becomes most apparent when envisioning the future role of occupational therapy in a particular setting or speciality. In encouraging students to look beyond current parameters, the role emerging placement opens up possibilities which may not emerge from a traditional clinical placement. Critically analysing the service from an occupational perspective enables the student to identify delivery gaps and formulate hypotheses about how an alternative service may seek to address these gaps, a process which is likely to involve some creative breaking of boundaries. One year on from the role emerging placement, skills and knowledge gained from the experience have been applied in clinical practice on numerous occasions. As a rotational Band Five Occupational Therapist currently working at a regional spinal injuries unit, there have been a number of opportunities:

1) to raise the issue of vocational rehabilitation,
2) to utilise change management strategies in formulating service development plans,
3) to initiate a timely and sustainable project within the constraints of the current service.

Vocational rehabilitation

When practising with clients of working age, care has been taken to ensure that issues of productivity are consistently addressed. This has involved liaison with clients' current employers, Disability Employment Advisors and advisors with Access to Work. On a more fundamental level, the Canadian Model of Occupational Performance (Law et al., 1996) has provided a frame of reference to enable consideration of each individual's unique motivation, or spirituality. With the understanding that positive expectations are critical to the achievement of positive outcomes (Krause & Pickelsimer, 2008), clients have been encourage to remain hopeful about maintaining their productive roles, including returning to work. The issue of vocational rehabilitation has also been addressed at a service-wide level through the delivery of an in-service presentation, which was later repeated at a mini-conference in the neighbouring regional spinal injuries unit. This presentation required research into current best practice and called for networking with other professionals. Knowledge of best practice at other units also inspired proposals for modifying the current occupational therapy service within the spinal injuries unit, with suggestions to be considered including the implementation of an outpatient clinic focusing on issues of productivity – a project which had recently been piloted at a neighbouring regional spinal injuries unit.

Change management

The role emerging placement afforded a valuable opportunity to reflect on effective change management principles. As a result, expectations for change have been carefully managed whilst on rotation. Complacency, or 'underestimating resistance to change', has been identified as one of the key mistakes made by those engaged in service development (Braveman, 2006, p. 202). As a result, any suggestions made for service development involved close consultation with both managers and colleagues across the multi-disciplinary team. An outpatient clinic involving Disability Employment Advisors from local job centres liaising with occupational therapists to provide support and advice on employment issues was an inspiring example of best practice – but it was not an achievable objective given the timeframe involved.

Sustainable project

Following discussion within the team regarding vocational rehabilitation opportunities, it was identified by the clinical lead that clients would benefit from an information pack containing useful contact details for agencies such as Access to Work, benefits advice lines, information on the Disability Discrimination Act and disability-focused driving assessments, and signposting to local employment services. This pack could also include information on accessible leisure facilities, charities such as the Spinal Injuries Association, and other community facilities. A project such as this was sustainable, realistic and achievable within the timeframe available. It is currently being undertaken with the input of an occupational therapy student on placement with the service.

Conclusion

Occupational therapy has a vital role to play in vocational rehabilitation services. But the profession should look towards expanding its boundaries in order to be able to deliver services which move beyond the welfare-to-work paradigm. Such services should involve interventions that are person-centred and reflect the individual's drive towards engaging in occupations that are meaningful to them and which impact positively on their health and well-being. This requires a wider understanding of the meaning of productivity, an understanding that includes, but is not limited to, paid employment.

For an occupational therapy student interested in vocational rehabilitation, a role emerging placement within a disability-focused employment service was an invaluable vehicle for developing skills, knowledge and ideas. The development of an occupationally focused project required careful reflection and effective communication, providing a unique opportunity to experience change management processes in practice. Critical analysis of the service combined with a wider reflection on the provision of vocational rehabilitation led to a deeper understanding of the welfare-to-work approach. This in turn led to the development of ideas about how an occupational perspective could enhance, and ultimately expand, current models of vocational rehabilitation. As advocated by Ross (2007, p. 234), what now remains is the resolve to "take these ideas forward and integrate them into our work with our clients". A role emerging placement not only provided an opportunity to develop the skills and knowledge needed to accept this challenge, it also ignited the passion to carry it out.

References

Alsop, A. (2004). Work matters. *British Journal of Occupational Therapy, 67* (12), 525.

Bisiker, J., & Millinchip, K. (2007). Developing a work rehabilitation project: 'Equal Pathways to Work'. *British Journal of Occupational Therapy, 70* (6), 259–263.

Black, C. (2008). *Working for a Healthier Tomorrow*. London: Department of Health. Available at: http://www.dh.gov.uk/en/Publicationsandstatistics/Publications/PublicationsPolicy AndGuidance/DH_083560. Accessed 1 January 2009.

Blesedell Crepeau, E., Cohn, E. S., & Boyt Schell, B. (2003). Occupational therapy practice. In E. Blesedell Crepeau, E. S. Cohn, & B. Boyt Schell, (Eds.), (*Willard & Spackman's Occupational Therapy* (10th ed.) (pp. 27–30). Philadelphia: Lippincott, Williams & Wilkins.

Blyth, B. (2006). *Incapacity Benefit reforms: Pathway to Work Pilots performance and analysis*. London: Department for Work and Pensions. Available at: http://www.dwp.gov.uk/asd/asd5/WP26.pdf. Accessed 24 September 2008.

Braveman, B. (2006). *Leading and Managing Occupational Therapy Services: An Evidence-Based Approach*. Philadelphia: F.A. Davis.

British Society of Rehabilitation Medicine. (2003). *Vocational Rehabilitation: The Way Forward* (2nd ed.). London: British Society of Rehabilitation Medicine.

College of Occupational Therapists. (2004). College of Occupational Therapists: Strategic vision and action plan for lifelong learning. *British Journal of Occupational Therapy, 67* (1), 20–28.

College of Occupational Therapists. (2007). *Occupational Therapy in Vocational Rehabilitation: A Brief Guide to Current Practice in the UK*. London: COT.

Department for Work and Pensions. (2002). *Pathways to Work: Helping People into Employment*. London: DWP. Available at: http://www.dwp.gov.uk/consultations/consult/2002/pathways/pathways.pdf. Accessed 9 June 2008.

Department for Work and Pensions. (2008). *Routes onto Incapacity Benefit: findings from a survey of recent claimants*. London: DWP. Available at: http://www.dwp.gov.uk/mediacentre/pressreleases/2008/mar/stat-040308.asp. Accessed 30 July 2008.

Finlay, L. (2004). *The Practice of Psychosocial Occupational Therapy* (3rd ed.). Cheltenham: Nelson Thornes.

Frank, A. O., & Sawney, P. (2003). Vocational rehabilitation. *Journal of the Royal Society of Medicine, 96* (11), 522–524.

Grahame, R. (2002). The decline of rehabilitation services and its impact on disability benefits. *Journal of the Royal Society of Medicine, 95,* 114–117.

Holmes, J. (2007). *Vocational Rehabilitation*. Oxford: Blackwell.

Jakobsen, K. (2004). If work doesn't work: How to enable occupational justice. *Journal of Occupational Science, 11* (3): 125–134.

Joss, M. (2002). Occupational therapy and rehabilitation for work. *British Journal of Occupational Therapy, 65* (3), 141–148.

Joss, M. (2007). The importance of job analysis in occupational therapy. *British Journal of Occupational Therapy, 70* (7), 301–303.

Kennedy-Jones, M., Cooper, J., & Fossey, E. (2005). Research article: Developing a worker role: Stories of four people with mental illness. *Australian Occupational Therapy Journal, 52* (2), 116–126.

Kielhofner, G. (2002) *A Model of Human Occupation: Theory and Application* (4th ed.). Philadelphia: Lippincott, Williams & Wilkins.

Krause, J. S., & Pickelsimer, E. (2008). Relationship of perceived barriers employment and RTW five years later: A pilot study among 343 participants with SCI. *Rehabilitation Counselling Bulletin. 51* (2), 118–121.

Law, M., Baptiste, S., McColl, M. A., Opzoomer, A., Polatajko, H., & Pollock, N. (1996). The person-environment-occupation model. A transactive approach to occupational performance. *Canadian Journal of Occupational Therapy, 63,* 9–23.

Lloyd, C., & Waghorn, G. (2007). The Importance of Vocation in Recovery for Young People with Psychiatric Disabilities. *British Journal of Occupational Therapy. 70* (2), 50–59.

Mercer, G. (2005). Job retention: A new policy priority for disabled people. In A. Roulstone, & C. Barnes (Eds.), *Working Futures? Disabled people, policy and social inclusion* (pp. 107–119). Bristol: The Policy Press.

Riddell, S. (2002). *Work Preparation and Vocational Rehabilitation: A Literature Review.* London: Disability Services Research Partnership. Available at: www.dwp.gov.uk/jad/2002/wae136rep.pdf. Accessed 23 June 2008.

Robdale, N. (2004). Vocational rehabilitation: the enable employment retention scheme, a new approach. *British Journal of Occupational Therapy, 67* (10), 457–459.

Ross, J. (2007). *Occupational Therapy and Vocational Rehabilitation.* Chichester: John Wiley & Sons.

Roulstone, A., & Barnes, C. (Eds.). (2005). *Working Futures? Disabled People, Policy And Social Inclusion.* Bristol: The Policy Press.

Royal College of Psychiatrists. (2002). *Employment Opportunities and Psychiatric Disability.* London. Available at: http://www.rcpsych.ac.uk/files/pdfversion/cr111.pdf. Accessed 29 July 2008.

Schonherr, M. C.; Groothoff, J. W.; Muder, G. A.; Schoppen, T. & Eisma, W. H. (2004). Vocational reintegration following spinal cord injury: expectations, participation and interventions. *Spinal Cord 42,* 177–184.

The Sunlight Trust. (2010). Available at: http://www.sunlighttrust.org.uk./ Accessed 18 October 2010.

Thurgood, J. & Frank, A. O. (2007). Work is beneficial for health and wellbeing: Can occupational therapists now return to their roots? *British Journal of Occupational Therapy, 70* (2), 49.

Townsend, E. A. (Ed.). (2002). *Enabling Occupation: An Occupational Therapy Perspective.* Ottowa: Canadian Association of Occupational Therapists.

Turner, A. (2002). Occupation for therapy. In A. Turner, M. Foster, & S. E. Johnson (Eds.), *Occupational Therapy and Physical Dysfunction.* Elsevier Health Sciences.

Waddell, G., & Burton, A. K. (2006). *Is Work Good for Your Health and Well-Being?* London: TSO.

Chapter 7

Promoting occupational therapy in a community health centre

Barry Trentham & Lynn Cockburn

Introduction: four villages, primary health care and the community health centre context

Recent policy directives acknowledge the necessity of establishing effective primary health care in order to maintain and improve population health (CSDH, 2008). It is therefore crucial that occupational therapists and their students become familiar with primary health care frameworks. This chapter outlines the community health centre (CHC) service delivery model in the province of Ontario and then describes current and potential roles for occupational therapists in these and emerging primary health care settings. It draws on our experience as two occupational therapists – former clinicians, currently educators and researchers – who worked as primary health care occupational therapists at the Four Villages Community Health Centre (FVCHC) in Toronto, Canada. We continue to be linked to the Centre and with the current occupational therapist through student fieldwork, collaborative research, and evaluation projects. In preparing this chapter we expanded on our work from a previous article published in 2007 in the *Canadian Journal of Community Mental Health* on the role of occupational therapists in primary health care and community development (Trentham et al., 2007).

Community health centres were developed across Canada in response to policy directives in the 1970s that outlined the need for a broader understanding of health to promote the health of Canadians. Federal documents, such as *Achieving Health for All: A Framework for Health Promotion* (Epp, 1986) and the Ottawa Charter on Health Promotion (WHO, 1986), provided the framework to develop CHCs. The need for increased resources for primary health care was further highlighted in the Romanow Commission Report (Romanow, 2002), *Building on Values: The Future of Health Care in Canada*. More recently, in the province of Ontario, a system of interdisciplinary primary care teams known as Family Health Teams (FHT) is being developed and include funded positions for occupational therapists. These teams provide a key entry point into comprehensive primary health care service delivery. Although they provide a range of traditional primary health care services, with the exception of the province of Quebec, only a few Canadian CHCs and FHTs currently provide occupational therapy services.

Role Emerging Occupational Therapy: Maximising Occupation-Focused Practice, 1st edition. Edited by Miranda Thew, Mary Edwards, Sue Baptiste and Matthew Molineux. © 2011 Blackwell Publishing Ltd.

Health promotion: The foundational guiding framework

The Ottawa Charter (WHO, 1986) sees health as, "a resource for everyday life, not the object of living" (p. 1). It defined health promotion as the process of enabling people to increase control over their health, and stated, "individuals or groups must be able to identify and realise their aspirations, to satisfy their needs, and to change or cope with their environment" (p. 1). The Ottawa Charter provided the framework from which to develop the occupational therapy primary health care service at the FVCHC. Fundamental to health promotion is an appreciation of the social determinants of health which include income, social status, social support networks, education, working conditions, physical environments, genetic endowment, personal health practices and health services (Minister of Supply and Services Canada, 1994; CSDH, 2008). The Ottawa Charter outlines several strategies to promote health that include building healthy public policy, creating supportive environments, strengthening community action, developing personal skills and reorienting health services (WHO, 1986). As advocated by leaders in health promotion, such as Best et al. (2003) and Raeburn and Rootman (1998), our work at the FVCHC offered a balanced approach to health promotion responding to broader, macro-level factors while also viewing individuals as agents able to control aspects of their own health.

Community health centres: The primary health care context

In this chapter, we follow the conventional distinction made between primary health care and primary care (Jeans, 1997; LeClair et al., 2005). Primary health care systems involve health professionals and others working together to deliver services in the context of the broader determinants of health such as education, workplaces and social participation (EICP in PHC Initiative, 2005). Primary care predominantly includes diagnosis, treatment and management of illness (LeClair et al., 2005). CHCs are non-profit, government-funded community organisations that provide primary health care for individuals, families and communities. In Ontario, CHCs are comprehensive and provide accessible service; are client- and community-centred; are made up of interdisciplinary teams that collaborate with other health and social services including schools, housing developments and workplaces; are grounded in a community development approach (AOHC, 2008) and anti-oppression and equity philosophies (Ministry of Health and Long Term Care, 2009). CHCs are governed by boards of directors elected by community members; the directors have responsibility for ensuring that the mandate of the CHC is fulfilled. The CHC staffing model is unique in that all staff are salaried including the physicians (as opposed to the usual form of fee-for-service physician remuneration). With more active physician involvement and a flattened hierarchical model, CHCs offer an effective team-based approach to service provision.

The FVCHC provides an example of a CHC that includes occupational therapy services. The FVCHC serves a culturally diverse population of approximately 70,000 people in the west end of Toronto, Canada. All socio-economic levels are represented in the community and in the client roster. Along with occupational therapy, the Centre has an interdisciplinary staff including nursing, medicine, social work, community health workers, nutrition, chiropody, physiotherapy and health promotion. Staff members are involved in community development, clinical service, health promotion and education, and interagency planning (FVCHC, 2009).

Occupational therapy at the Four Villages Community Health Centre

Although a client would not necessarily require a medical diagnosis to use the services of the occupational therapist, the majority of the occupational therapy clients at the FVCHC are people living with disabilities and chronic illness including mental health challenges. Given the diversity of health problems experienced by FVCHC clients, CHC occupational therapists by necessity are generalists, a distinctive characteristic of primary health care occupational therapists found in other countries (Aas & Grotle, 2006). Primary health care occupational therapy in CHCs requires balancing community and population perspectives with the enablement of occupational development for individual participants. This is a complex set of skills to manage. This section describes how the occupational therapist role blends attention to several levels of service provision within the primary health care context. Occupational therapy interventions in CHCs span the community development continuum proposed by Jackson et al. (1989). These interventions build from an initial focus on individual health issues and one to one casework aiming to develop individual capacities, to mutual support and group programming for those with similar issues, to collective, advocacy and social change activities which aim for participation, control of services and the strengthening of social movements.

Often marginalised individuals, including those living with disabilities, connect first with the occupational therapist who may become the primary health care provider. Alternatively, other team members refer clients with perceived occupational limitations to the occupational therapist directly. Though the occupational therapist addresses the source of the initial referral – often related to specific self-care activity limitations – additional assessment is focused on the skills, abilities, and knowledge that the individual has to offer. This process reflects a community capacity building approach to occupational therapy delivery further elaborated on in the following text.

Occupational therapy responding to individual occupational issues and health needs

The occupational therapist at FVCHC works with individuals on a client-centred, one-to-one basis, using accepted occupational therapy processes and models (e.g. Townsend & Polatajko, 2007). Specifically, these have included: chronic illness self-management education, splinting, adaptive equipment and technologies, wheelchair assessment and training, home safety assessment and adaptations, psychosocial counselling and support, pain management, vocational assessment, housing advocacy, and assistance with long-term care assessments and placement. The occupational therapist must become aware of individual skills, and the supportive and disabling social conditions affecting each client, in order to achieve the client's desired occupational outcomes. Although the initial presenting issue may be addressed, the occupational therapist in this primary health care setting has a broader view in considering how the individual client can benefit from and contribute to various group-based health promotion strategies.

Linking individuals with opportunities for occupational engagement through group programmes

One of the goals of the occupational therapists working at FVCHC has been to identify the strengths, capacities and skills inherent in different client groups and communities. The combination of individual and group programming leads to numerous connections and opportunities between individuals and their communities. Some of these opportunities will be within the Centre, while others will be outside the Centre in the local community. The training and ability to blend individual and group perspectives with a focus on occupational engagement and the outcome of social participation is unique to the occupational therapist role. By encouraging users of the FVCHC to see themselves as members of, and contributors to, the community, the occupational therapist begins to address the impact of occupational deprivation on health and looks for ways to develop individual capacities by linking to existing occupational opportunities. The group programmes at FVCHC are largely made up of people with varying abilities and life experiences. Young and old, able-bodied and disabled, new Canadians and well-established citizens participate in health-promoting activities together. As is unique to an occupational perspective, the focus is not necessarily aimed at the amelioration of disability or illness but on improving quality of life through the enablement of occupational engagement and participation.

The process of developing new group programmes starts with the Centre's strategic planning and community surveys. Individual users of the Centre also provide input into programme planning, viewed by the occupational therapists as a health-promoting occupation in itself. The ability to do programme planning inclusively with people of diverse abilities and backgrounds requires an occupational therapist with strong facilitation and enabling skills. The importance of such skills are often not initially appreciated by students and other team members but are crucial for the effective implementation of enabling strategies with groups (Table 7.1).

A rehabilitation perspective is infused in much of the group work. For example, the *Getting on with Life and Its Challenges* programme aims to promote health and coping skills. Some participants may feel that they are in a rehabilitation or recovery process, and that participating in the group is part of their rehabilitation, while others may perceive it to be part of their ongoing personal growth and development. Linking clients with community organisations and groups requires significant time and skill. To maintain and initiate these partnerships, the occupational therapists link with key players in the community and may attend tenant or community organising events, participate in seniors' coalitions or consumer run support groups and connect with business improvement associations. The

Table 7.1   Current and past examples of group programmes offered at FVCHC.

Getting on with Life and its Challenges	• Mental health support and skill development programme • The occupational therapist works with a steering committee to develop, plan and organise workshops • Discussions, developing skills, building friendships and sharing information; the group has engaged in participatory research projects addressing occupational engagement and occupational deprivation (Reid, 2008)
Sharing Food Cultures	• Planning and preparing of meals; joint programme with the nutritionist • Older adults living with disabilities, many of whom immigrated to Canada many years ago, with younger new immigrants and refugee families • Participants learn from each other about food and life in Canada • Some members from this programme developed catering small business
Community Action Group	• Advocacy for a more senior-friendly neighbourhood • A group of seniors, most of whom lived with illness or disability • Over time the group developed partnerships with other seniors' advocacy groups and became active in lobbying for senior friendly changes to transportation, health benefits and health service provision
Chetwynd Community Development Group	• Several social and health agencies with young families living in social housing • The aim was to foster social connections between neighbours and providers, and to then identify shared issues and solutions. • As part of this multi-year project, the occupational therapist along with other providers planned and facilitated linkages during a week-long outdoor camp setting
Kids Can Create Programme	• A joint programme with nursing, dieticians and occupational therapists • Focus on children and promoting fine-motor development of young children • Used creative food-related activities to increase cooking and nutritional knowledge
Expressive Arts Therapy	• A joint social work and occupational therapy programme • Aimed at assisting women to improve their ability to express themselves through art-based activities
Women's Self-Esteem Group	• A joint social work and occupational therapy psychosocial education programme • Aimed at supporting women who self-identify as having low self-esteem • Some participants are living with a mental health diagnosis
Seniors Wellness Group	• Originated as a joint walking programme; developed into a weekly exercise, wellness education and support programme • Partnership with the occupational therapist and a public health nurse • For seniors living with chronic and significant physical disabilities and illness. Participatory planning and evaluation processes were incorporated into the design allowing for participant control and meaningful engagement in the programme

FVCHC recognises that some of the occupational therapists time must be dedicated to this aspect of work and that not all of the occupational therapists work is individually focused.

Going broader: The CHC occupational therapist as a systemic change agent

Beyond individual and small group-based enabling strategies, occupational therapists and their students working at CHCs bring a system-wide perspective. Systemic change is required to overcome the lack of available occupational opportunities experienced by many clients. Systemic change requires engagement in political processes associated with social action approaches to community development (Rothman & Tropkin, 1987), an aspect of practice only recently being explicitly discussed within occupational therapy (Pollard et al., 2008; Leclair et al., 2005), and one that would seem to be a necessary area for professional development if we are to be true to the goal of occupational justice. For example, transportation costs, access barriers and perceived discriminatory eligibility criteria for adapted transportation were repeatedly viewed as barriers to greater community participation needing to be addressed.

Occupational therapy programmes aimed at broader community level issues were viewed as important as the health and occupational enablement needs of individuals. Clearly, these different levels of intervention interact and inform each other. occupational therapists are well placed to bridge the gap between these environments from different sectors. For example, community actions taken on by the Community Action Group, such as sidewalk curb cuts, equitable transportation advocacy and the installation of benches, enable the occupational performance of a group of individuals while benefiting a larger group of community members. At the same time, individual level interventions such as time management strategies and interpersonal skills enable individual citizens living with disabilities or chronic health issues to participate in such community-building occupations.

Lessons learned: Reflections on 15 years of occupational therapy at FVCHC

When writing a chapter such as this one offers an opportunity to reflect on our work as primary health care providers and to raise questions about possible reasons for the relative invisibility of occupational therapist contributions within the primary health care environment. We provide suggestions for occupational therapy to better position itself within primary health care and to identify opportunities for occupational therapists and their students to become more involved in CHCs and other primary health care venues. Occupational therapy frameworks share the perspective promoted by primary health care advocates. Primary health care principles speak to the need to respond to the health needs of populations, neighbourhoods and communities at both individual and broader systemic levels using strategies that consider the social determinants of health. Occupational therapy would seem to be a natural fit, yet often the public is not aware of this aspect of occupational therapy work. Given this clear fit between the ideals and practice of occupational therapy and primary health care practice settings, why has there not been more of an occupational therapy presence in the primary health care arena? There is no single answer nor is there a body of literature to respond to this question, however, based on our experience, we offer some possible reasons. Acknowledging the limitations of these speculations, some thoughts and working hypotheses are shared with the aim of stimulating discussion, research and action.

Coupling evidence with good stories that resonate with the public

Currently relatively little research exists on the roles and evidence for occupational therapy in primary health care contexts such as CHCs. Though it may be assumed that this is the primary reason for the lack of occupational therapy advancement in this area, lack of evidence is only part of the story. Many of the services that are provided within CHCs are provided by non-regulated health and social-service providers who do not necessarily have a strong record of evidence-based practice. For example, health promoters, community development workers and early childhood workers are professional groups that may be included on CHC teams.

It could be argued, however, that many of the strategies employed by these service providers are in fact grounded in research evidence. For example, there is a growing body of evidence that supports the need for programmes that respond to the social determinants of health, such as early childhood enrichment, programmes aimed at the amelioration of poverty, adequate housing and social support network development (CSDH, 2008). Currently, no one discipline can claim full ownership over these broad level strategies. Funding decisions may be more focused on what is done through health promotion strategies and programmes, and not on which discipline provides the service. Although evidence may play a role at higher policy levels in mandating the array of service providers available at the primary care arena, its role may be overestimated in marketing efforts.

CHCs are governed by community boards which provide direction for service delivery in keeping with government guidelines and mandates. Community boards are to be responsive to the unique health care needs of the various communities within their geographical regions. Although the Ontario Ministry of Health and Long Term Care outlines a list of potential service providers, each CHC is afforded some flexibility in selecting the array of services to be provided. The decisions made by community members who advise their CHCs on human resource decisions are arguably seldom based on rigorous reviews of the evidence-based literature. Rather, we would suggest that decisions are often made based on the public awareness of services that have been provided in the past, such as medicine and nursing and, importantly, on good public interest stories about the benefits of various conventional and complimentary service providers.

The public may not be aware of the holistic and alternative perspective that occupational therapy offers; a perspective that can make significant contributions to health, wellness, and primary health care. Other professions such as physical therapists, chiropractors, naturopaths, art therapists, and yoga instructors may offer a more ready image of the nature of their healing powers and health-promoting approaches than occupational therapy. Stories highlighting the role of many of these health professions are more evident in public discourse. Daily newspapers and health and wellness magazines are more likely to write about the claimed benefits of these services than about occupational therapy. Bold claims are made by numerous non-regulated health care providers who market themselves successfully as holistic healers. These providers have captured the attention of a public disheartened with conventional medical approaches to service delivery. The public seems hungry for providers who work with them as partners to improve their health and use the language and concepts of holistic health. Occupational therapists need to use more marketable stories aimed at a broader public in the places where they learn about health, such as newspapers, wellness magazines and health fairs.

Articulating the added benefit of occupational therapy

A number of other service providers have a relatively long history working with populations and communities to respond to the social determinants of health. For example, most CHCs employ social workers, community health workers, community development workers and health promoters. Many of these providers view their primary health care role as building the capacity of communities and populations to create healthy communities through such strategies as community capacity building, social support network building, improved housing and anti-poverty advocacy. It is hard to argue that occupational therapists have a similar track record using these strategies. Occupational therapists are often more costly than other providers. What then is our added cost-benefit? We believe that the unique skill set and broad, holistic occupational perspective adds significant benefit to a CHC team.

　　At the FVCHC, we often bridged the gap between the more medical or individualistic perspective of the nurses and doctors to the community and environmental focus of health promoters and community development workers. Unlike the holism offered by alternative care providers which remains centred on the individual body, the holistic vision of occupational therapy goes beyond the body–mind–soul tricotomy to embrace and intervene through contexts and environments. From an occupational therapy perspective, whole bodies are seen as part of the larger social whole; bodies and their abilities to do and engage in the world are shaped by the environments in which people live, work and play. Often seen as a liability in medical institutional settings, the generalist and broad, ecologically informed holistic vision of health from an occupational perspective needs to be marketed to what is becoming a more knowledgeable and consumer savvy population. The time is ripe for a public that demands an alternative to non-holistic health care.

Challenging medical hegemony over the primary health care discourse

One further impediment to an expanded role within primary health care relates to how the discourse of primary care and primary health care is controlled. Although definitions of primary care and primary health care have been articulated (Jeans, 1997; LeClair et al., 2005), it has been our experience that, in common parlance, there remains a lack of clarity (Haggerty et al, 2007; MOHLTC, 2009). Very often discussions about primary health care service delivery are reduced to or are assumed to be about primary medical care provided by medical doctors or nurse practitioners. This hegemonic tendency sidelines and suppresses the potential contributions of other primary health care practitioners including occupational therapy.

Though it could be said that many private practice occupational therapists, for example, those who work with children, in counselling roles or in a variety of community organisations, are working in primary health care, they often do not define their roles as such. Occupational therapists working in such settings could frame this work as primary health care and challenge limited, taken-for-granted definitions. A useful example of this strategy comes from Manitoba. The Manitoba Society of Occupational Therapists (Leclair et al., 2005) produced a document which clearly links primary health care and occupational therapy. It was written specifically to foster the development of occupational therapy in a particular context. It also calls for the development of remuneration and organisational models that are equitable and allow for providers to practice according to primary health care principles.

Similarly, we need to be vigilant as to when occupational therapy regulatory bodies, professional associations or educational programmes limit occupational therapy potential in primary health care in the manner in which the role of occupational therapy is articulated, regulated and marketed. Promotional materials including visual images (which are the key vehicles through which our stories are told) should consider vignettes and images that convey the role of occupational therapists working in various contexts from individual service provision to group, community and government levels. For example, to facilitate marketing efforts, occupational therapy educational programmes and service organisations often promote themselves along with physical therapy and speech language pathology as rehabilitation providers. This is a term that public policy makers understand. It can serve us well. At the same time, however, it may inadvertently hide what occupational therapy has to offer in primary care and primary health care settings. The broader, holistic, ecologically based perspective described above is not often a shared framework amongst rehabilitation workers. Physiotherapists work with individuals, and for the most part specifically with their bodies. Occupational therapists work with individuals and their surroundings in context. By marketing ourselves as rehabilitation providers, we may advance our situation in hospital sectors, but block further progress in community and primary health care settings.

Working towards sustainability

The sustainability of programmes such as those described above necessitates the development of better evaluation tools, and policies that recognise the complexity and time needed for the establishment and maintenance of effective partnerships with health and social-service providers as well as informal community associations (e.g. religious groups, tenant associations). Existing assessment and evaluation tools available to occupational therapists for the most part are focused on individual level outcomes and interventions.

Students need to be exposed to a broader array of group and community level assessment tools that effectively track efforts aimed at building community capacity to respond to community health issues. (e.g. Hancock & Minkler, 1997; McKnight & Kretzmann, 1997)

Broadening descriptions of who we serve

We had to rethink how our client base was described. At FVCHC, disability and the need for rehabilitation, while one possible aspect, were not the only criteria for service provision. It is not uncommon for an occupational therapist, using a primary health care orientation, to be working with clients where the aim is to promote health or to prevent illness, such as young unemployed persons or well seniors. Neighbourhood safety and wellness support groups aim to prevent injuries and promote positive mental health while enabling engagement in community-building occupations; members do not necessarily have a diagnosable illness or disability.

An occupational perspective differentiates the occupational therapist role from other health professionals whose focus is on treating impairments, illness or disease. An occupational perspective has the potential to create a seamless integration of community development principles. The occupational therapist's attention to inclusion and accessibility, including abilities to work with people with disabilities, can mean that they are able to find unique ways of linking key players in the community.

Infusing an occupational justice perspective to the CHC

Thinking of the programme initiatives outlined above as community occupations that enhance community health and well-being illustrates the challenges of a practice that is based on occupational justice principles. The programmes respond to occupational marginalisation, alienation, imbalance or deprivation. Occupational therapy programmes in the CHC setting can have significant impact on the occupational lives of many individuals, directly or indirectly. Whether through increased opportunity to participate in inclusive, meaningful and socially valued community occupations, feelings of connectedness to others in their community, or through measures in the physical environment to increase safe community mobility for older adults, these programmes aimed beyond individual level change to change outcomes at the community and, to a lesser extent, policy levels.

However, as occupational therapists we appreciate how privileged we have been to work within a health organisation that values and supports community-focused health change. CHCs are unique and few in number. The majority of community and institutionally based health care settings provide remuneration only for the provision of interventions aimed at individuals living with illness or disability. Although community occupational participation of people living with chronic illness and disability is often blocked due to socio-environmental barriers (e.g. inaccessible transportation systems, poverty, stigma), occupational therapists are prevented from fully responding to these barriers because such strategies may be viewed by those in decision-making roles as outside the health professional's role. This is an example of the problem of being categorised within the same rehabilitation category as physiotherapy.

Occupational therapists interested in reframing practice from an occupational justice perspective could benefit from linking the growing understanding of the determinants of occupational participation and occupational enablement to the language, concepts and strategies of primary health care, the social and environmental determinants of health, human rights, health promotion and illness prevention.

Opportunities for greater occupational therapist involvement

CHCs rely on community volunteers to implement, guide and advise primary health care programmes. Numerous opportunities exist for occupational therapists and their students to contribute through such volunteer programmes. For example, CHCs are governed by community boards. Occupational therapists interested in community health and primary health care can become members of a CHC and seek membership on the board. At the FVCHC, occupational therapists not employed by the Centre were invited to share their insights with other CHC staff and with client groups. Occupational therapists could take advantage of opportunities to market their expertise to CHC staff and board members with the aim of providing fee-for-service, time-limited contractual consultative or workshop educational experiences, and in doing so demonstrate the potential of an occupational therapy perspective. For example, one occupational therapist volunteered her time to provide a workshop on promoting health through everyday occupations to community groups.

Distinct from, though similar to, CHCs with their primary health care mission is the evolving health care delivery model known as Family Health Teams (FHT). The province of Ontario has recently listed occupational therapist as one of the approved and funded health professions to be included on these teams. The FHTs provide primary care using an interdisciplinary team consisting of physicians, nurses, nurse practitioners, nutritionists and others depending on the decisions made by groups of providers. Occupational therapy expertise in working with people with chronic mental and/or physical illness and disability is a particularly attractive skill set for FHTs, given the time needed for work with individuals with such complex health needs. Occupational therapists are also advised to market their proven track record in supporting these individuals to self-manage their health and occupational challenges. Though not fully established, the role of the FHT occupational therapist may be more limited in community development scope compared to that of CHC occupational therapists.

The growing demand for the interdisciplinary focus of FHTs and CHCs may in part be related to the current and increasing complexity of an aging population. It is well known that people are living longer, many with a complexity of medical and mental health issues (WHO, no date). There are increasing demands on an already stretched hospital and long-term care system. Policy directives that aim to build alternative models of care for older adults in order for them to age in place are becoming more common. For example, Ontario's Aging at Home strategic direction funds innovative interdisciplinary programmes to support older adults in their homes. Health challenges related to use of technology, accessibility, home safety, social support, innovative housing initiatives and health promotion have been examples of funded initiatives. Occupational therapists should respond to the call for such proposals.

Occupational therapy educators can stimulate the creativity and energy of students to think about innovative practice areas assignments and fieldwork experiences. Students should have opportunities to hear about and become familiar with primary health care organisations such as CHC and FHTs. Though there is an ongoing debate about role emerging placements (e.g. Cooper and Raine, 2009), it is crucial for development in primary health care that the risks of these kinds of placements be addressed so that students and supervisors can be supported in benefiting from them. Occupational therapy educators and researchers could mentor students and therapists who are interested in primary health care and community development and to engage in collaborative research partnerships. Student occupational therapists can also combine learning while making valuable contributions to programme evaluation and research (Reid et al, 2008).

Conclusion

This chapter provides a description of the role of primary health care occupational therapy in one CHC in Toronto, Canada. The variety of services provided by the occupational therapist at FVCHC requires a generalist approach that considers the occupational and health challenges of individuals and communities. The ecologically based and broad holistic occupational perspective offered by occupational therapists fits well with the aims of primary health care. The CHC environment provides one practice context where this perspective can be fully realised.

Occupational therapy is well placed to provide leadership in further developing primary health care delivery. However, the occupational therapy profession must be better able to market its contributions to the public and to policy decision makers if it is to become more prominent. Occupational therapy educators and primary health care occupational therapists can support occupational therapy student engagement in this area of practice through CHC–University evaluation and research partnerships, supporting emerging field-work placements and providing students with the language, tools and perspectives needed to take on leadership roles within this emerging practice area.

References

Aas, R., & Grotle M. (2006). Clients using community occupational therapy services: Sociodemographic factors and the occurrence of diseases and disabilities. *Scandinavian Journal of Occupational Therapy*, *14* (3), 150–159.

Association of Ontario Health Centres (AOHC) (2008). *Who we are and what we do*. Available from http://www.aohc.org/aohc/index.aspx?CategoryID=71.

Best, A., Stokols, D., Green, L. W., Leischow, S., Holmes, B., & Buchholz, K. (2003). An integrative framework for community partnering to translate theory into effective health promotion strategy. *American Journal of Health Promotion*, *18*, 168–176.

Cooper, R., & Raine, R. (2009). Role-emerging placements are an essential risk for the development of the occupational therapy profession: the debate. *British Journal of Occupational Therapy, 72* (9), 416–418.

CSDH Commission on Social Determinants of Health. (2008). *Closing the Gap in a Generation: Health Equity Through Action on the Social Determinants of Health. Final Report of the Commission on Social Determinants of Health.* Geneva: World Health Organization.

Enhancing Interdisciplinary Collaboration in Primary Health Care Initiative. (2005) *The Principles and Framework for Interdisciplinary Collaboration in Primary Health Care.* Available from http://www.eicp.ca/en/principles/documents.asp.

Epp, J. (1986). *Achieving Health for All: A Framework for Health Promotion.* Ottawa, ON: Health and Welfare Canada.

Four Villages Community Health Centre (FVCHC), (2009). http://www.4villageschc.ca/.

Haggerty, J., Burge, F., Lévesque, J-. F., Gass, D., Pineault, R., Beudieu and Santor, D. (2007). Operational definitions of attitrubes of primary health care: consensus among Canadian experts. *Annals of Family Medicine, 5* (4), 336–344.

Hancock, T. & Minkler, M. (1997). Community health assessment or healthy community assessment. In: Minkler, M. (Ed.), *Community Organizing and Community Building for Health* (pp. 139–156). New Brunswick: Rutgers University Press.

Jackson, T., Mitchell, S., & Wright, M. (1989). The community development continuum. *Community Health Studies, 13* (1), 66–73.

Jeans, M. E. (1999) Primary care and primary health care for an integrated system. *Healthcare Papers, 1* (1), 33–36.

Leclair, L., Restall, G., Edwards, J., Cooper, J., Stern, M., Soltys, P., & Sapacz, R. (2005). *Occupational Therapists and Primary Health Care.* Available from http://www.msot.mb.ca/uploads/PositionPaper_PrimaryHealthCare.pdf.

Minister of Supply and Services Canada, (1994). *Strategies for population health: Investing in the health of Canadians. Prepared by the Federal, Provincial, and Territorial Advisory Committee on Population Health for the meeting of the Ministers of Health*, Halifax, Nova Scotia, September 14–15, 1994. Ottawa, ON: Health Canada.

Ministry of Health and Long Term Care (2009). Community Health Centres. *Community Health Centres.* Available from http://www.health.gov.on.ca/english/public/contact/chc/chc_mn.html.

McKnight J., & Kretzmann, J. (1997). Mapping community capacity. In; Minkler, M. (Ed.), *Community Organizing and Community Building for Health* (pp. 157–174). New Brunswick: Rutgers University Press.

Pollard, N., Sakellariou, D., & Kronenberg, F. (Eds.). (2008). *A Political Practice of Occupational Therapy.* Edinburgh: Elsevier Science.

Raeburn, J., & Rootman, I. (1998). *People-Centred Health Promotion.* West Sussex, UK: John Wiley and Sons Ltd.

Reid, N. Cockburn, L., Shin, J., Ashton, B., Nowakowski, A. Smith, S., & Wall, B. (2008, November). *Mental Health Consumers' and Occupational Therapists' Responses to a Calendar about Occupational Engagement.* Poster presented at the CAMH: Building Equitable Partnerships Symposium 2008, Toronto, Ontario.

Romanow, R. (2002). *Building on values: The future of health care in Canada.* Retrieved November 25, 2005, from http://www.hc- sc.gc.ca/english/pdf/romanow/pdfs/HCC_Final_Report.pdf.

Rothman, J. & Tropkin, J.E. (1987). Models of community organization and macro practice perspectives. In: F. M. Cox, J. L. Erlich, J. Rothman, & J. E. Tropman (Eds.), *Strategies of Community Organization* (4th ed.; pp. 26–63). Itasca: Peacock Publishers, Inc.

Townsend, E. A., & Polatajko, H. J. (2007). *Enabling Occupation II: Advancing an Occupational Therapy Vision for Health, Well-being, & Justice Through Occupation*. Ottawa: CAOT Publications ACE.

Trentham B., Cockburn L., Shin J. (2007). Health promotion and community development: An application of occupational therapy in primary health care. *Canadian Journal of Community Mental Health*, *26* (2), 53–70.

World Health Organization (WHO). (1986). *Ottawa Charter for Health Promotion*. Health Promotion, 1, iii–v.

WHO (no date). *Older people and primary health care*. Retrieved November 5, 2009, from: http://www.who.int/ageing/primary_health_care/en/index.html.

Chapter 8

Occupational therapy: Making a difference to people with cardiac failure in the community

Emma Brown & Barbara Gurney

Introduction

Promoting community-based occupational therapy can be a difficult task within certain areas of practice and specialty. Partly borne out of confusion regarding the occupational therapist's role, but also because within the UK there are few occupational therapists working directly within essentially community-based primary care teams where many chronic conditions are managed. Community cardiac services are one such example. Further, many cardiac services are geared towards those people who have experienced heart attacks or acute episodes of cardiac pathology. Whereas heart failure is a common, debilitating syndrome the prevalence of which increases markedly with age, prognosis is poor and symptoms such as breathlessness, fatigue and fluid retention cause significant functional problems and impede the person's ability to perform the daily occupations of life. The emphasis of heart failure care is a medical one in order to slow disease progression and control symptoms. There is limited focus on improving quality of life and/or function. With the global concern regarding the aging population, and associated costs to society, the emphasis of current cardiac care should be on maintaining health and well-being by keeping people active and independent for as long as possible. Encouragement of healthy lifestyle habits such as regular exercise, normal body weight and healthy eating can significantly improve the risk of developing heart failure or improve the long-term prognosis.

Currently, occupational therapists have limited involvement in community-based cardiac teams within the UK, and are more likely to be found in cardiac rehabilitation services. With their skills in promoting and supporting people to engage in meaningful occupation and emphasis on improving function and quality of life, occupational therapists have a lot to offer the care of people with heart failure. There is currently a lack of research evidence as to the benefit of occupational therapy involvement within heart failure care. This chapter reflects a role emerging placement in a community cardiac service by an occupational therapy student, which highlights how an occupational perspective and role could enhance the service for people with cardiac failure. There are case examples of the occupational therapy intervention carried out with this particular client group, which

Role Emerging Occupational Therapy: Maximising Occupation-Focused Practice, 1st edition. Edited by Miranda Thew, Mary Edwards, Sue Baptiste and Matthew Molineux. © 2011 Blackwell Publishing Ltd.

should prove useful for those practitioners who wish to follow a similar route. It also demonstrates the value and variety of interventions that an occupational therapist could offer within this area.

Heart failure: the facts

Heart failure is a common, debilitating syndrome. The prevalence of heart failure is estimated to be between 2 and 3% and rises sharply at the age of 75 years or more, with a prevalence at ages 70 to 80 years between 10 and 20%. The aetiology most commonly associated with the term 'heart failure' is coronary heart disease (myocardial infarction, arrhythmias in particular, Atrial Fibrillation), hypertension and cardio-myopathies. Toxins (alcohol being the most common) and endocrine causes such as diabetes, hypothyroidism and hyperthyroidism are also a feature (Box 8.1).

Symptoms that cause functional problems are, most notably, dyspnoea (shortness of breath), fatigue and fluid retention; the latter can be so severe in the legs as to significantly reduce mobility (Box 8.1). Often patients in the advanced stages of the disease process develop significant weight loss with muscle wasting, further impeding the ability to perform daily activities of life (Poole-Wilson & Ferrari, 1996). Typically, prior to referral and engagement into cardiac rehabilitation services in the community, people with a diagnosis of heart failure pass through a variety of medical tests and investigations. These usually include regular ECGs, blood tests and a definitive diagnosis following investigation with an ECHO (echo-cardiogram).

The diagnosis of heart failure is graded into four classifications listed below (adapted from Chavey et al., 2001):

- Class I: no symptoms on ordinary physical activity
- Class II: slight limitation of physical activity by symptoms
- Class III: less than ordinary activity leads to symptoms
- Class IV: inability to carry out any activity with symptoms.

Prognosis is poor for those with heart failure and figures vary vastly, with a 5-year mortality varying from 26 to 75% (Cowie et al., 1997), obviously, those who present with symptoms of a higher classification of the disease tend to have a poorer prognosis.

Box 8.1   Definition of heart failure (Dickstein et al., 2008)

Heart failure is a clinical syndrome in which patients have the following features:
- Symptoms typical of heart failure
  - Breathlessness at rest or on exercise, fatigue, tiredness, ankle swelling.
- Signs typical of heart failure
  - Tachycardia, tachypnoea, pulmonary rales, pleural effusion, raised jugular venous pressure, peripheral oedema, hepatomegaly.
- Objective evidence of a structural or functional abnormality of the heart at rest
  - Cardiomegaly, third heart sound, cardiac murmurs, abnormality on the echocardiogram, raised natriuretic peptide concentration.

Heart failure accounts for 5% of cardiac medical admissions to hospital and as with many chronic conditions re-admission and the 'revolving door syndrome' for these patients is common (Horton, 2005). Increasingly, therefore, services have developed significantly into the community-based, nurse-led heart failure services such as the one in which an occupational therapy perspective was included. Evidence suggests that programmes involving community specialist nurse management can improve health outcomes in patients with heart failure (Blue et al., 2001; Stromberg et al., 2003; Stewart & Blue, 2004) and ultimately reduce hospital admissions. Although such communities are classed as a 'nurse led' service, it should be remembered that a multidisciplinary approach is needed to ensure patients receive an excellent standard of care (Sochalski et al., 2009). However, the focus of many aspects of heart failure care is a medical one with titration of medicines being the objective for many services. It is known that medications such as ACE inhibitors and beta blockers are recommended as a mainstay of treatment, as they extend life (National Institute for Clinical Excellence, 2005). There is less research and less emphasis on using non-medical treatments to improve quality of life (Peters-Klimm et al., 2009), although there is some evidence that there is a direct correlation between perceived improved quality of life and improved mortality in cardiac failure patients (Juenger et al., 2002). Ultimately, as with cardiac rehabilitation, it is necessary to consider the person needs holistically beyond that of medical and nursing care and this requires delivery by a multi-disciplinary team approach.

Occupational therapy within cardiac services

Tackling coronary heart disease (CHD) is a UK government priority, with the National Service Framework (Department of Health, 2000) and National Institute for Clinical Excellence (NICE) guidelines (Royal College of Physicians, 2003) setting standards for service provision within cardiac rehabilitation and heart failure. Highlighted within these standards is the need for cardiac care to be delivered by a multidisciplinary team as these programmes improve patient's quality of life, satisfaction with care and the risk of unplanned hospitalisation. Despite this, Lewin et al. (1998) investigated adherence to cardiac rehabilitation guidelines within the UK and found that of 273 cardiac rehabilitation programmes, less than half had an occupational therapist within the team. No corresponding data relating specifically to heart failure care and occupational therapy appears evident. Within the UK, occupational therapists are more likely to be found in cardiac rehabilitation programmes rather than in heart failure care (NICE, 2009), and there is little research evidence generally concerning the role of occupational therapy within cardiac services. The literature that exists illustrates that occupational therapy intervention has traditionally been focussed on teaching stress management and relaxation techniques (Tomes, 1990; Tooth & McKenna, 1996). It can be argued that these are generic skills which can be undertaken by any health care professional and are essentially not taking advantage of the unique skills of occupational therapy. The provision of specialist equipment, grading and adapting occupations, fatigue management and task simplification, as well as relaxation and stress management programmes can be common occupational therapy interventions within cardiac services (Doherty, 2003). Helm and Ellison (1988) evaluated an occupational therapy programme which included education around their condition and a graded leisure activities session providing the opportunity to practice normal everyday activities in a protected environment. Participants found the practical aspects of the occupational therapy programme to be particularly useful. This research is clearly outdated and there is sparse contemporary evidence to support occupation-focused occupational therapy within community cardiac services and specifically with people with chronic heart failure.

Occupational therapy within cardiac care should focus on promoting the pursuit of purposeful, meaningful occupation in daily life in order to maximise functional performance and minimise de-conditioning (Oliver & Sewell, 2003). This includes increasing activity tolerance and promoting reintegration into desired occupations within established activity limitations (Doherty, 2003). Research has shown that participating in occupations that are meaningful to the individual leads to improved function, subjective well-being and life satisfaction (Clark et al., 1997; Law et al., 1998). In addition, increased engagement in physical, social and productive activities has been found to reduce mortality rates in the elderly population (Glass et al., 1999). For people with a cardiac condition, enhancing a person's opportunity and ability to participate in occupations of importance to them could potentially lead to an increased quality of life and improved health. Occupational therapy interventions should target the symptoms of breathlessness and fatigue that affect occupational performance, and it is important to assess the person's view of their quality of life and mood, as these are known to be poor in people with heart failure (Tattersal, 2005). More research is needed to ascertain the role of occupational therapy within cardiac services, particularly within community teams and within the care of cardiac failure.

Occupational perspective of cardiac services

An occupational perspective is based on the premise that humans are occupational beings, who experience and express their sense of self-worth and identity through occupation (Wilcock, 1998). Through engagement in occupations, a person's physical, mental and social needs and capabilities are met. There are arguments that suggest that susceptibility to illnesses may arise as a result of occupational deprivation, alienation or imbalance, factors that can either be a cause or consequence of illness (Wilcock, 1998; Whiteford, 2000). Living with a heart condition can have a profound impact on a person's life and on the lives of their family and friends (Oliver & Sewell, 2003). Occupational imbalance occurs when engaging in occupations fails to meet physical, emotional and social needs (Wilcock, 1998). Conversely, having an equal balance of physical, mental, social and rest occupations contributed to a sense of well-being and perceived good health (Douglas, 2006). With the case of CHD and specifically a progressive condition such as heart failure, people may not be able to experience a balance of health-giving occupations, for fear of exacerbating symptoms or increasing the chance of experiencing another cardiac event. Cardiac patients often report that they are afraid of restarting activities and interests which they enjoyed before their heart condition, and they get used to being unable to carry out certain activities (Helm & Ellson, 1988). This fear and anxiety may promote behavioural avoidance as a coping strategy and reduce physical functioning due to a sense of inadequacy in performing activities of daily living (Doering et al., 2004; Dunderdale et al., 2007). The desire to perform daily activities can be heavily outweighed by the effort required; therefore, insufficient time may be spent engaging in occupations that they want to do and the majority of time spent on the things they have to do. Depression can be common and the adjustments people are required to make to their lifestyle are a constant reminder of their clinical condition (Oliver & Sewell, 2003). People with heart conditions often withdraw from particularly physically strenuous occupations and social contact, spending the majority of their time in sedentary occupations, ultimately leading to further de-conditioning decreased fitness and consequential worsening of symptoms. By adopting an occupational perspective and understanding of some of the occupational issues associated with heart failure can help identify underlying causes of concern and explore ways of improving occupational performance; thus bringing a different approach to the treatment of people with conditions such as heart failure.

An overview of community cardiac care in the community

One of the main occupational issues which seem to face individuals with a heart condition is building up activity tolerance levels and confidence to be able to resume some of the activities they used to do before their cardiac episode. Heart failure patients in particular can experience significant problems in resuming occupations due to the chronic and progressive nature of their condition, with symptoms such as fatigue and breathlessness impacting on their ability to carry out occupations (Stewart & Blue, 2004). Fatigue symptoms can dramatically hinder daily life activities or occupations and the consequences of fatigue can further exaggerate the experience of engaging in them (Falk et al., 2007). People with heart failure currently receive little in the way of rehabilitation and can potentially lead predominantly sedentary lifestyles. The community cardiac setting provides an opportunity to consider this particular client group, by understanding the impact symptoms of heart failure have on their ability to carry out everyday occupations and identifying strategies to enable them to get back to doing the occupations of importance to them. This was primarily achieved in a role emerging placement within a community-based cardiac service, through the application of fatigue management strategies, examining lifestyle factors impacting on energy levels and by grading and pacing activities (Thew & Pemberton, 2008). Increasing engagement in occupations which are health giving, potentially leads to improved health, well-being and quality of life. Falk et al. (2007) found that restorative activities, such as appreciation of nature, fishing, gardening and social events, were helpful in alleviating some of the symptoms of fatigue. In addition, keeping active prevents de-conditioning of the muscles which increases fatigue levels and can lead to worsening of symptoms.

Two cases of heart failure are described to illustrate how an occupational perspective delivered a more multidisciplinary and holistic approach to clients who were receiving care from a community cardiac team. Both were initially interviewed and assessed within their own homes. The assessment tools used with these clients included the 'Minnesota Living with Heart Failure' questionnaire (Rector & Cohn, 2008), to measure quality of life and gain a baseline score before intervention. The Model of Human Occupation interest checklist was employed to gather information on a client's strength of interest and engagement in a number of activities in the past, present and future, focussing particularly on leisure interests. In addition, the life and energy jug analogy (Thew & Pemberton, 2008) was utilised to identify occupations that were draining, boring, stimulating, frustrating or stressful for a person; and activity diaries were used to indicate how the clients occupied their time and performed certain occupations (Thew & Pemberton, 2008). The interest checklist and life jug analogy were adapted for use with this particular client group. Interventions focussed on using problem solving, grading and pacing, and fatigue management techniques to assist clients to re-engage with or pursue meaningful occupation. The following case study examples illustrate the work carried out with the two clients.

Case study 1

Mrs Jones is 42–year-old housewife with heart failure and lives with her husband and teenage son. Her main symptoms include fatigue and breathlessness, which have a significant impact on her energy levels and ability to carry out every day activities such as gardening, cleaning and going out. The occupation that she really wanted to get back to doing was country walks. She reported having to take frequent rests, and described the difficulties and frustration she had adjusting to this. In addition, she often tried to do everything at once if she was having a good day, resulting in her feeling tired for the next day or two. She tended to do everything in the morning when her energy levels were higher and was often tired by the afternoon, frequently requiring a short nap. The majority of her time was spent doing housework leaving little time and energy for pleasurable activities.

   The purpose of the occupational therapy intervention was to try and help her maximise her energy levels during the day using fatigue management strategies and to encourage more pleasurable activities within her weekly schedule, to create energy. Principles of grading and pacing were used to suggest ways of increasing her tolerance levels to gradually getting back to the things she wanted to do. For example, walking, by decreasing the pace and distance of walks or doing three short walks over the week rather than one long walk at the end of the week, could enable her to gradually increase her tolerance levels to perform this occupation more effectively. The client engaged well with some of the fatigue management principles discussed during sessions, and began to make some changes to her lifestyle. She changed her routine to do the laundry in the evening and over two days rather than in the morning on one day. This had no impact on her fatigue levels and gave her some free time during the day to do something else. This particular client seemed to be struggling to accept her condition and the fact that she could no longer do things the way she used to do. This needed to be taken into account whilst working with her as there was a risk that she could potentially start withdrawing from activities due to fear of failure or not being able to perform them to her satisfaction.

Case study 2

Mrs Smith is a 68–year-old female who lives on her own in a warden-controlled flat. She has mobility difficulties, using a scooter to get around, and her main symptoms were breathlessness and fatigue associated with her diagnosis of class III heart failure. The client reported feeling tired all the time and not having the energy to do things and stated how fed up she was at feeling this way all day, every day. She believed the increase in her fatigue levels was due to her condition worsening. The main occupation she engaged in was watching TV; however, she also did all the housework, played bingo with a friend, visited the local town on her scooter, and socially engaged neighbour and residents in the communal area. The one occupation that she wanted to re-engage with (which she had stopped over the last two years) was going to the market in the centre of the city. Although this was something she really wanted to do, she felt strongly that she could not due to her poor mobility and symptoms of her condition. In this instance, using a problem-solving approach and providing means of overcoming some of the barriers to be able to get into and around town worked really well. This included providing links to support agencies such as specialist bus services, mobility equipment and 'motability' services. The client was also given advice regarding grading the occupation, and she was thinking of going with her granddaughter during the school holidays. Breaking down barriers and introducing small achievable incremental changes is important in giving people the motivation and confidence to engage in occupations they may have felt unable to do.

Working occupationally with this client group

The focus of the occupational therapy intervention was to support heart failure patients to identify individual strategies to enable them to resume or pursue meaningful occupation. The above case studies illustrate the differing needs of two clients with a similar heart condition, emphasising the need to work in a client-centred manner focussing on occupations which are important to them and their lifestyle. The first client required help and support adjusting her lifestyle to be able to perform occupations she wanted or was required to do, within her activity limitations. The second client led quite a sedentary lifestyle, requiring more support in identifying occupations of interest, and problem solving to help overcome some of the barriers for her to engage in occupations of importance to her. The assessment tools used proved valuable in gathering detailed information around occupations of interest to the clients and how occupations they currently participated in were performed. This assisted in targeting the intervention in order to facilitate occupational engagement for both clients. The Interest Checklist is particularly useful if people are struggling to identify occupations of interest. Other assessment tools that can be used by occupational therapists involved with heart failure care include the Assessment of Motor and Process skills (Fisher & Kielhofner, 1995), Canadian Occupational Performance Measure (Law et al., 2005) and Hospital Anxiety and Depression scale (Zigmond & Snaith, 1983; Tattersal, 2005). The Hospital Anxiety and Depression scale (HAD) scale was already used by the specialist nurses within this cardiac service. However, the Canadian Occupational Performance Measure (COPM) examines satisfaction with occupational performance in the areas of self-care, productivity and leisure and is designed to detect change in self-perception of occupational performance over time, making this tool a useful outcome measure.

There is no current research evidence concerning the utilisation of any occupational therapy assessment tools within cardiac care; however, the COPM has been proven to be effective with a wide variety of disabilities and ages (Law et al., 2005). A brief questionnaire was sent out to each client to provide feedback following the interventions and therapeutic visits. All clients stated that they were treated with respect and felt listened to. In addition, they thought the role of occupational therapy and purpose of the visits were clearly explained; and they found the sessions useful. Evaluation is an essential part of the occupational therapy process and should be carried out after a significant period of time has lapsed to allow time for interventions to have an effect, although this more longitudinal measure was not made.

Overall, this placement has demonstrated that there is considerable potential input that occupational therapy can make to this particular area of cardiac care, and brought an extra dimension to an already highly skilled team of nurse specialists. Heart failure, in particular, is an area where there is limited occupational therapy contribution currently, particularly in community settings; however, occupational therapists can play a significant role in enabling people with heart conditions to lead active and occupational lives without fear of exacerbating their symptoms.

Heart failure service perspective

The role emerging placement demonstrated the benefits of occupational therapy provision to a community-based heart failure service in a large city in the UK. The team of experienced heart failure and cardiac rehabilitation nurses had some misconceptions when first approached regarding the placement. These stemmed from the nursing teams collective experience of occupational therapy which appeared to concentrate on limited personal care (e.g. dressing assessments) for usually, those in inpatient settings (e.g. recovering from a Cerebral Vascular Accident). Some nursing staff had also experienced working with occupational therapists in cardiac rehabilitation settings, but only in respect to stress and anxiety management. These misconceptions of the limited role of occupational therapy were dispelled by students being directly placed in community cardiac teams. They were able to explain and to some degree demonstrate that occupational therapy can have a broader application, which concerns increasing functionality by seeing humans as 'occupational beings'. Clients with heart failure were considered for the first time to be experiencing poor levels of occupational performance, and significant loss of occupational roles and function due to the nature of the disease process. Fatigue as a major symptom of heart failure particularly in stage III and above, along with medication, side effects in particular, beta blockers, which reduces energy and hence can make many feel unable to perform even the most basic of tasks.

An issue which all cardiac clients appear to face is the inability to recognise the need to goal set and pace themselves, and although all the cardiac nurses are skilled in offering support for their clients around goal setting and pacing, it is often difficult to allocate sufficient time to work in this way, as the focus is often and necessarily on medication management and palliative care. In addition, cardiac nurses do not consider skills such as fatigue management and grading activity or occupations as a core skill, whereas it appears other professionals such as occupational therapists have these skills taught within their basic professional curricula.

Although more research is required as to the true benefit of an occupational therapy allocation to community cardiac services particularly with clients diagnosed with cardiac failure, it has appeared to the team that there is a benefit to the development of such a role. Clearly, the two case studies demonstrated here are insufficient evidence; however, both clients clearly derived found some benefit from the occupation focused interventions that were carried out by the occupational therapy student.

The potential and future of occupational therapy within this type of setting

Heart failure has a significant impact on a person's life, with symptoms such as fatigue and breathlessness making it difficult to carry out normal everyday occupations. The impact of heart failure on a person's life may be related as much to the psychological adaptation to the disease as to impairment in physical functioning (Tattersal, 2005). Both the National Service Framework for Coronary Heart Disease and NICE guidelines highlight the need for a multidisciplinary programme of secondary prevention in heart failure to reduce the risk of subsequent cardiac problems and promote return to a full and normal life (Department of Health, 2000; Royal College of Physicians, 2003). Occupational therapists have an important role to play in the assessment and treatment of people with heart failure due to their holistic approach and focus on engagement in meaningful occupation to promote health and well-being (Tattersal, 2005). Additional core skills of occupational therapists include assessment of the environment, expert knowledge of equipment and adaptations, assessment of functional potential, problem solving and grading and pacing (College of Occupational Therapists, 2004). Occupational therapists can therefore play a significant role in assisting people with heart failure to make a positive adjustment to their condition, and can add to the quality and improvement to a person's functional ability in the areas of self-care, productivity and leisure (Tattersal, 2005). Traditionally, the occupational therapists role within areas of cardiac care has focused on equipment, relaxation and stress management, within hospital settings. The government's white paper 'Our Health Our Say: A New Direction FOR Community Services' sets out the future of health services to be provided outside the hospital and in more local convenient settings, including the home (Department of Health, 2006). Long-term conditions that are well managed in the community means emergency bed days are diminished considerably. This chapter has offered a small, but useful demonstration of the potential contribution occupational therapy can make to people with heart failure within their homes. Occupational therapists should seriously consider embracing the opportunity to make a difference within these community-based teams, utilising their skills in promoting occupational function and performance. More research is needed to examine the potential contribution occupational therapists can make to areas such as cardiac failure care. By adopting an occupational perspective, there is a potential role for occupational therapists to tap into some of the issues faced by individuals with cardiac conditions, in terms of supporting people to engage or re-engage in the occupations they used to, need to or are required to do.

Conclusion

The need for intensive multidisciplinary care for people with cardiovascular diseases has long been recognised. Living with a cardiac condition such as heart failure can have a significant impact on an individual's ability to carry out everyday occupations. By focussing on promoting reintegration into desired occupations or the pursuit of meaningful occupation, within established activity limitations, people can lead healthy and fulfilling lives. With the political and current global concern regarding the aging population, more people are living for longer with heart failure, but ultimately without improvement in daily occupational performance, this could be a clear and costly burden to society. With greater emphasis on improving the amount that someone with cardiac failure can do, as well as improving psycho-social morbidity, the relative costs can be reduced.

Current treatment of people with a heart condition centres on improving function, increasing quality of life and supporting people to resume a full a life as possible, clearly a role the nursing team play an integral part. Occupational therapists can greatly contribute to this by concentrating on the health providing nature of engaging in meaningful occupation. Although this example, of two case studies and the experience of a student within a community cardiac team, can hardly offer a legitimate source of research, what is clear is that there are misconceptions amongst cardiac teams about the role and what potential occupational therapists can offer. The nurses learnt from the students' occupational perspective, that not only did they have some of their misconceptions around the traditional role of the occupational therapist challenged but they also had the importance of goal setting and pacing or grading occupations reiterated to them.

Recent research has identified that restorative activities can be helpful in alleviating some of the symptoms of fatigue in heart failure patients, clearly a role in which occupational therapy can play a vital part. However, more research is needed to assess the potential contribution occupation can make within cardiac care, and the specific nature of restorative activities that can be beneficial or health providing for people with chronic heart failure and other cardiac conditions. There is clearly a need to focus on occupations that are meaningful to the client, highlighting the need for an individual, client-centred approach. Obviously whilst the benefit of occupational therapy involvement is critically lacking in terms of research-based evidence, a possible way forward would be to introduce a skill-mix to a cardiac team with outcome measures in terms of frequency of admissions, subjective quality of life measures and costs in relation to the amount of services required to support that person. With the increased focus of health services and treatments being provided in the community, occupational therapists should consider embracing new and developing roles, where they can apply their unique skills in promoting and supporting engagement in meaningful occupation as integral to maintaining or attaining health and well-being.

References

Blue, L., Lang, E., McMurray, J. J., Davie, A. P., McDonagh, T. A., Murdoch, D. R., Connolly, E., Norrie, J., Round, C. E., Ford, I., Morrison, C. E. (2001). Randomised controlled trial of specialist nurse intervention in heart failure. *BMJ (Clinical Research Ed.). 323* (7315), 715–718.

Chavey, W.E 2nd, Blaum, C.S., Bleske, B.E., Harrison, R.V., Kesterson, S, & Nicklas, J.M. (2001). Guideline for the management of heart failure caused by systolic dysfunction: Part I. Guideline development, etiology and diagnosis. *American Family Physician. 64* (5), 769–774.

Clark, F., Azen, S. P., Zemke, R., Jackson, J., Carlson, M., Mandel, D., Hay, J., Josephson, K., Cheey, B., Hessel, C., Palmer, J., Lipson, L. (1997) Occupational therapy for independent-living older adults: a randomised control trial. *Journal of the American Medical Association, 278* (16), 1321–1326.

College of Occupational Therapists (2004) *Definitions and Core Skills for Occupational Therapy.* London: COT.

Cowie, M. R., Mosterd, A., Wood, D. A., Deckers, J. W., Poole-Wilson, P. A., Sutton, G. C., Grobbee, D. E. (1997). The epidemiology of heart failure. *European Heart Journal. 18* (2), 208-225.

Department of Health, (2000). *National Service Framework for Coronary Heart Disease.* London: Department of Health.

Department of Health, (2006). *Our Health, Our Care, Our Say: A New Direction for Community Services.* London: Department of Health.

Doering, L., Dracup. K., Caldwell, M (2004) is coping style linked to emotional states in heart failure patients? *Journal of Cardiac Failure, 10*, 344—349.

Doherty, R.F. (2003) Cardiopulmonary dysfunction in adults. In: E. B. Crepeau, E. S. Cohn, & B. A. Boyt-Schell (Eds.), *Willard and Spackman's Occupational Therapy* (10th ed.). London: Lippincott, Williams & Wilkins.

Douglas, F. M., (2006). Occupational balance: the relationship between daily occupations and wellbeing. *International Journal of Therapy and Rehabilitation, 13* (7), 298–301.

Dunderdale, K., Furze, G., Thompson D. R., Beer, S. & Miles, JNV. (2007) Health-related quality of life from the perspective of patients with chronic heart failure. *British Journal of Cardiology, 14*, 207—212.

Falk, K., Granger, B. B., Swedberg, K., & Ekman, I. (2007) Breaking the vicious circle of fatigue in patients with chronic heart failure. *Qualitative Health Research, 17*, 1020–1027.

Fisher, A., & Kielhofner, G. (1995). Skill in occupational performance. In G. Kielhofner(Ed.), *A Model of Human Occupation: Theory and Application* (2nd ed.). Baltimore: Williams and Wilkins.

Glass, T., De Leon, C., Marottoli, R., & Berkman, L. (1999) Population based study of social and productive activities as predictors of survival among elderly Americans. *British Medical Journal, 319*, 478–483

Helm, M., & Ellison, J. (1988) Cardiac rehabilitation: occupational therapy enhancement of an existing cardiac outpatient rehabilitation programme. *British Journal of Occupational Therapy, 51* (11), 385–389.

Horton R. (2005). The neglected epidemic of chronic disease. *Lancet, 366* (9496), 29–31.

Juenger, J., Schellberg, D., Kraemer, S., Haunstetter, A., Zugck, C., Herzog, W., Haass, M. (2002). Health related quality of life in patients with congestive heart failure: comparison with other chronic diseases and relation to functional variables. *Heart, 87*, 235–241.

Law, M., & Canadian Association of Occupational Therapists. (2005). *Canadian Occupational Performance Measure.* Toronto: CAOT–ACE.

Law, M., Steinwender, S., Leclair, L. (1998) Occupation, health and well-being. *Canadian Journal of Occupational Therapy*, *65* (2), 81–91.

Lewin, R. J. P., Ingleton, R., Newens, A. J., Thompson, D. R. (1998). Adherence to cardiac rehabilitation guidelines: a survey of rehabilitation guidelines in the United Kingdom. *British Medical Journal*, *316*, 1354–1355.

NICE. (2005). *Chronic Heart Failure. National Clinical Guidelines for Diagnosis and Management in Primary and Secondary Care.* The National Collaborating Centre for Chronic Conditions. London: NICE. *5*: 1–163.

NICE. (2009) *Specifying a cardiac rehabilitation service* [internet] Available from [Accessed August 2009].

Oliver, K., & Sewell, L. (2003). Cardiac and respiratory disease. In: A. Turner, M. Foster, & S. E. Johnson (Eds.), *Occupational Therapy and Physical Dysfunction*. London: Churchill Livingstone.

Peters-Klimm, F., Campbell, S., Müller-Tasch, T., Schellberg, D., Gelbrich, G., Herzog, W., Szecsenyi, J. (2009). Primary care-based multifaceted, interdisciplinary medical educational intervention for patients with systolic heart failure: lessons learned from a cluster randomised controlled trial. *Trials*, *10*, 68.

Poole-Wilson, P. A., & Ferrari, R. (1996). Role of skeletal muscle in the syndrome of chronic heart failure. *Journal of molecular and cellular cardiology.* (*28*) :2275–2285.

Rector, T. S., & Cohn, J. N. (2008) Minnesota Living with Heart Failure questionnaire. Available from: http://www.mlhfq.org/ [accessed 21/06/08].

Royal College of Physicians. (2003). NICE Guidelines No. 5 – *Chronic Heart Failure – National Clinical Guideline for Diagnosis and Management in Primary and Secondary Care.* London: Royal College of Physicians.

Sochalski, J., Jaarsma, T., Krumholz, H. M., Laramee, A., Mcmurray, J. J. V., Naylor, M. D., Rich, M. W., Riegal, B., Stewart, S. (2009). What works in chronic care management: the case of heart failure. *Health Affairs, 28* (*1*), 179.

Stewart, S., & Blue, L. (2004). *Improving Outcomes in Chronic Heart Failure: Specialist Nurse Intervention from Research to Practice.* London: BMJ.

Stromberg, A., Martensson, J., Fridlund, B., Levin, L. A., Karlsson, J. E., & Dahlstrom, U. (2003). Nurse-led heart failure clinics improve survival and self-care behaviour in patients with heart failure. *European Heart Journal*, *24* (11), 1014–1023.

Tattersal, K. (2005). Heart failure. In: A. McIntyre, & A. Atwal (Eds), *Occupational Therapy and Older People.* Oxford: Wiley Blackwell.

Thew, M. & Pemberton, S. (2008). Energy for life. In: M. Thew, & J. McKenna (Eds.), *Lifestyle Management in Health and Social Care.* Oxford: Blackwell Publishing Ltd.

Tomes, H. (1990) Cardiac rehabilitation: an occupational therapist's perspective. *British Journal of Occupational Therapy*, *53* (7), 285–287

Tooth, L. & McKenna, K. (1996) Contemporary issues in Cardiac Rehabilitation: Implications for Occupational Therapists. *British Journal of Occupational Therapy*, *59* (3), 133–138.

Whiteford, G. (2000). Occupational deprivation: global challenge in the new millennium. *British Journal of Occupational Therapy, 63*, 200–204.

Wilcock, A. A. (1998) Occupation for health. *British Journal of Occupational Therapy, 61* (8), 340–344.

Zigmond, A. S., Snaith, R. P. (1983) The hospital anxiety and depression scale. *Acta Psychiatrica Scandinavica, 67* (6), 361–70.

Chapter 9

Community development

*Deborah Windley**

Introduction

This chapter explores part of the wealth of opportunity that awaits occupational thera-pists within the broader and less traditional sectors of our communities. Experiences of occupational therapy students with refugees, older adults and people with mental health issues are recounted, revealing rich roles for occupational therapists working directly with referred clients as well as in establishing environments within agencies and institutions that are conducive to enabling engagement in occupation and community participation. The chapter demonstrates via narratives from the students, the occupational therapists over seeing the placements and the on-site educators, the richness of learning that took place and the impressions the students and their projects left.

Community development

Community development focuses upon empowering people to gain control over the con-ditions in which they live. At its core reside a set of values that embrace social justice, self-determination, working collectively, equality and justice, reflection, participation, political awareness and sustainable change (Department for Communities and Local Government's Community Empowerment Division, 2006). These principles have been strongly influenced by the work of Paulo Friere and the concept of 'conscientisation'; this refers to the development by marginalised people of critical awareness skills which en-ables them to reflect upon the social reality of their situation (Freire, 1972) This awareness can become the catalyst for empowerment:

> *the process by which disadvantaged people come together to increase their control over events that control their lives . . . . goal is to enable communities, families and individuals to read and transform their reality . . . . . . Empowerment, democracy and community participation should be judged by the extent to which they are participating in activities they have to determine for themselves.* (Kaseje, 1991)

*With contributions from Ann Day, Leeds Library Service, Sharon Witton, SROT; Jacinta Houlihan, SROT; Jess Adcock, SROT; Jasmine Littler, SROT and Kayley Cookson, SROT.

Role Emerging Occupational Therapy: Maximising Occupation-Focused Practice, 1st edition. Edited by Miranda Thew, Mary Edwards, Sue Baptiste and Matthew Molineux. © 2011 Blackwell Publishing Ltd.

This definition is of direct relevance to occupational therapists who are concerned with facilitating access to meaningful occupation for groups and communities.

Occupational justice

The concepts of occupational justice and occupational risk factors (Townsend & Wilcock, 2003) have been applied to create a framework and a language through which occupational therapists can legitimise and articulate their interest in and contribution to the issues of social justice and inequality. The profession has long understood the relationship between the person, their environment and occupation (Yerxa, 1998), yet traditionally occupational therapists have addressed primarily contextual barriers when treating individual health conditions.

Occupational risk factors emerge from barriers to engagement with occupation due to environmental factors. Occupational imbalance (Townsend & Wilcock, 2003, p. 253), deprivation (Whiteford, 2004) apartheid (Kronenberg & Pollard, 2005) and alienation (Wilcock, 1998), p. 257) result from inequalities in access to resources, or other limitations in the ability to engage and participate in a way that is meaningful and fulfilling. Wilcock (1998) has explored the relationship between these risk factors and pre-clinical conditions such as boredom, anxiety, sleeplessness and low self-esteem which can lead to clinical health concerns such as depression, substance abuse, obesity and cardio-respiratory conditions. Poverty is the most wide-reaching factor preventing equal access to resources and occupational choices. The relationship between poverty and poor physical and mental health is well documented by Annandale (2003). The cycle of poverty is sustained further through the poor social infrastructure which accompanies poor communities. The resultant lack of choice and self-determination lead to further helplessness and powerlessness, so that opportunities such as education are seen as meaningless and irrelevant (Narayan et al., 2000). Where whole communities suffer occupational injustice through lack of access to meaningful employment, education and social resources, the results can be seen potentially in anti-social behaviour, poor health outcomes and wasted potential (Whiteford, 2004). The challenge for the occupational therapy profession is whether this cycle can be broken through occupational engagement, and enablement of communities to overcome some of the environmental restrictions which limit human potential (Whiteford et al., 2000).

Cultural change

Occupational therapy has begun to explore not only the restorative value of occupation but also how engagement and participation in occupation can contribute to the growth and development of communities (Watson, 2004). The development of community psychology as a sub-discipline of psychology is useful for understanding how a health profession can make the cultural change required to work within a community development model of practice. Whilst psychology traditionally focussed on the individual or the micro-system of family and peers, community psychologists adopted a more ecological perspective focussing on the macro-socio-political structures. Community psychologists have made oppression their primary concern, rather than individual behaviour. From this perspective, maladaptive behavioural choices can be understood as adapting as well as one can to oppressive and stressful circumstances. Their concern is to examine the root causes of issues and promote competence and well-being through self-help, empowerment, community development and social and political action by moving away from intervention which places the cause of the psychological issue within the individual to be treated (Nelson & Prilleltensky, 2005).

The concept of occupational justice suggests a similar need for a broader macro perspective to occupational therapy practice. Furthermore, an occupational perspective can empower individuals through involvement in personally significant occupations by developing skills and self-confidence through engagement.

Community Development as a focus of role emerging placements: the Leeds Metropolitan University experience

Students' studying to become occupational therapists at Leeds Metropolitan University, must complete a six-week role emerging placement in a setting where occupational therapists currently do not practice. Some of the services have a community development focus to their work providing an opportunity to explore the potential for occupational therapy in these settings. The students experiencing these placements are not expected to *practice* occupational therapy but to identify how an *occupational perspective* can contribute to the service and develop a sustainable project which utilises this perspective. The following case studies use the experience of students on placement in two of these settings: an initial accommodation site for asylum seekers and a city wide library service, to explore the potential of an occupational perspective in furthering community development and tackling social exclusion.

Case study 1: working with asylum seekers

This narrative draws upon the experience of two groups of two students over two years. The students worked with the Refugee Council, a voluntary organisation focused upon supporting and assisting asylum seekers and refugees in the United Kingdom (UK). The Refugee Council is contracted by the UK Government to provide briefings to asylum seekers about the asylum and dispersal process (Refugee Council Online, 2010). The students were based in an initial accommodation site the details of which are explained below.

The context

Individuals can apply for asylum under the United Nations (1951) Convention and protocol relating to the status of refugees at their port of entry into the UK. After an entry screening process they are taken to an initial accommodation site in order to arrange for a solicitor to manage their case and set an interview date for their asylum claim (Refugee Council Online, 2010). They have a right to remain in the country until a decision is made on their asylum application. They are ineligible for any benefits and forbidden to work until they are granted refugee status by the UK Home Office (Gower, 2009). This particular setting accommodates over 200 newly arrived asylum seekers who remain there between 3 to 4 weeks until they are dispersed into the community. All individuals and families have a shared bedroom and are provided with their food and drink at set meal times. The Refugee Council attempts to provide services in addition to the briefings by developing and running groups and other activities; however, this aspect of their work is not funded.

Restart Skills for the UK

The first occupational therapy students on this placement established 'Restart Skills for the UK', a programme which focused upon cooking, shopping and budgeting, using local transportation and other resources with an introduction to basic English language skills required for these tasks. A kitchen in a local community centre run by the primary care (NHS) trust was made available to the programme. The resulting session plans and information were left as a legacy to enable the programme to be run by project workers and volunteers since professional staff were not part of the budgeted complement on site.

The occupational therapy practice placement educator perspective

The occupational therapy practice placement educator, Sharon Witton supervising the students in their role emerging placement, was also working at that time for the Refugee Council, although not in her designated professional role. She had a previous interest in and commitment to this population which led her to assume another role co-ordinating the 'Talks Team'. This project enabled asylum seekers to have access to meaningful occupation through talking about their experiences to the British public and educating them about the realities of life as an asylum seeker and refugee. As Sharon explains:

> The 'Restart Group' developed the notion of what is meaningful and purposeful. They focussed on what was culturally relevant for the group members . . . They had considered and been open to the need to make the sessions have individualised meaning. Some people were focussed on the opportunity to learn English in the context of an activity. For others 'Restart' gave the chance to link past and present occupational history. There was a really poignant moment in one session where the person whose menu was cooked, tasted the food and her eyes filled up. I think that is a credit to the students' facilitation, that link of the cooking and the flavours, enabled her to access something from her past.

Sharon spoke about the fractured nature of the process around seeking asylum often necessitating leaving home precipitously, leaving individuals in a state of shock. Therefore, any situation, however slight, that provides a chance to reconnect with the familiar, such as "cooking and eating a familiar meal is significant". 'Restart' encouraged those who may have felt isolated to share a mutual experience through a shared activity. The people come from different cultures, countries and backgrounds. The lack of shared language and restricted opportunity for engagement frequently results in feelings of isolation and being unable to gather to share experiences. 'Restart' also encouraged newly arrived asylum seekers to access British culture and institutions through shopping and cooking. "The UK asylum process holds people in a bubble outside British society and culture, with the centres designed as self contained units where people are not actively encouraged to engage with one another". Consequently this undermines further the individual's self-confidence. "I see this intervention as a radical act as the students challenged this position by facilitating engagement with British culture".

There is evidence that mental and physical health often deteriorates two or three years after asylum seekers arrive (Burnett & Fassil, 2000). It is suggested that this could be a result of a lack of control and choice over personal lives and decisions, hostile and sometimes abusive treatment by others, and being exposed to poverty and poor housing conditions. The most important psychological issue is 'loss' of family, country, occupation, house, status, identity, self-esteem, health, well-being and all things familiar (Burnett & Peel, 2001). As Sharon continued:

> *The asylum process does damage people . . . We need to think about what we need to offer to facilitate the transition better. People in this situation are often traumatised and unable to make plans for their future. Occupational therapists' philosophical commitment to engaging in something meaningful as a pre-cursor to well being and the ability to look at the component parts of activity to develop skills and promote participation means there is a role for occu-pational therapists in these settings. However, the asylum system is a holding system whereby you are not part of Britain at all, so you are not entitled to your rights until you get permission to stay. So I'm very cynical that there could be an investment in the health of asylum seekers beyond the basics.*

Using occupation science-based evidence, they made it possible for others to understand all of this too and thus enabled the submission of a proposal that resulted in a successful funding bid for the programme.

Social and activity space

The second group of students were placed in the same initial accommodation site discussed above. They chose to focus upon the physical environment and address the way in which this had become a barrier to occupation. Feelings of isolation, boredom, lack of control and choice are prevalent amongst this client group impacting on both physical and mental health; two thirds of refugees have reported anxiety or depression at some time (Burnett & Peel, 2001). The period awaiting a decision about their status may be, and often is, an extremely gruelling and difficult time for an asylum seeker (Tribe, 1999). There were three aspects to this project: changing the intimidating and unwelcoming environment of the TV room which was the only communal space for activity providing access to basic resources to help adults and children fill their time; and developing a resource list of local individuals and organisations able to provide useful input to facilitate occupation in the future.

The student perspective

People in that setting were so occupationally deprived, they had nothing to do on a daily basis and by providing something to engage with we felt it would have an effect on their health and well being. We brought an occupational perspective by highlighting that all human beings have a need to do things on a daily basis and shouldn't be excluded from that because they have left their country of origin. Some of the staff were consumed in their role with the briefings and missed the fact that some people are really bored and the consequences of that. Whereas we went in thinking about what people are doing with their time. We wanted to create opportunity for participation and realised there needed to be a change in the environment to facilitate engagement.

From the outset, Jess and Jacinta, recognised the impersonal nature of the environment, with some rooms remaining locked, nothing going on and no apparent encouragement for any activities or events to take place. The residents tended not to leave the premises due to lack of finance, motivation and need to be available to attend briefings. Once the renovations of the leisure space were underway, comments were heard regularly that the atmosphere was changing. More active participation between clients was visible, with more women now entering the space and the television not necessarily being the centre of attention at all times. Families started to sit together, which created a much warmer and less intimidating context from previously when only men populated the room. There were opportunities to observe more casual and relaxed behaviours, revealing more of the clients' personalities than was readily displayed during formal meetings and briefings.

When we were redecorating and cleaning clients were queuing up to help and the staff said that they had no idea how much people were willing to help and be involved. The centre manager noted the change in the atmosphere in the building. People were not just hanging about in the corridor and sitting on the ground but using the room. I think the staff came to realise what the value of 'doing' gave to people. There are a number of services working for this client group and we realised that we needed to get all of these on board to make an impact. We wanted to build up partnerships with the services so that when we left they had a list of others who could help maintain opportunities for occupation.

One of students' aims was to connect with the local community to reveal a population that they rarely see.

The centre is so excluded and isolated from the community. When I first went there I asked in a local shop around the corner where it was and they had no idea. I suppose as there is such stigma around refugees and asylum seekers the services avoid publicity. But I think if they brought these people more into the community, so that people understood what they have been through, it would help both the community and the asylum seekers. It would help aid transition and integration into the community and start to breakdown stigma and fear. We had wanted to publicise locally what we were doing and encourage community participation but the organisation feared it would attract negative attention which may have been the case if it appeared that one group was getting extra resources.

Jess and Jacinta ran a session with the staff on site eliciting ideas about how the project could be sustained once the students were not available. After this session, once ideas had been voiced, the staff began to exude a sense of ownership for the project. They began to discuss possible activities and events that could be organised and the roles they could play to make it happen. Sustainability planning of this nature is critical to ensure that an innovation of this type will continue in some form. While the students had planned to leave programme plans and ideas behind once they did leave, the notion of the ideas coming from the staff was much more palatable.

> *What I realised at the end was the value of enabling and encouragement; instead of giving and telling, encouraging and showing people and letting them do it themselves; Not just holding groups but changing the environment making it possible for people to do what they please. That is what occupational therapy is about, not doing things for people but enabling.*

Case study 2: community development within a library service

This narrative draws on the experience of two groups of two students over two years, who were on placement with the Leeds library service.

The context

The role of libraries in the UK has evolved greatly and they are now seen as providing the focus for communities, acting as a repository for local resources. Libraries are involved in many aspects of community development with contributions to agendas related to social inclusion through promoting lifelong learning and also promoting health and well-being. The service seeks actively to increase access, encouraging communities to identify how libraries can help to meet their needs. There is an emphasis on targeting 'hard to reach' communities and working on developing partnerships. The library service in Leeds has 53 static libraries and a large mobile library resource.

The occupational therapy student contribution

The first two students on placement within the service focussed upon reducing barriers and thereby facilitating access to the library for isolated older adults. The students devised a series of sessions designed to enable participants to engage in and share personal reminiscences using the library's extensive archives, books and audio-visual material. Detailed session plans and resources were left for the librarians to implement once the occupational therapy students were not on site. Part of the aim of the group was to familiarise the participants with the resources and equipment available for current as well as future use. Hopefully, this would ensure that the service will continue and the participants will continue to attend once this group was concluded. The second pair of occupational therapy students developed a similar package from the first to be implemented by library staff; however, their focus was on the needs of people with enduring mental health needs living in the community. They developed a creative writing group 'A Way with Words', as the central occupation.

The on-site practice placement educator perspective

The on-site practice placement educator (Ann Day), was initially sceptical about what occupational therapy could contribute to the service:

> *My knowledge of occupational therapy prior to these placements was based on personal experience with my Mum when she came out of hospital, around equipment and the occupational therapist trying to get her to go to pottery classes which she hated. So I was originally worried about the idea of occupational therapy students with the service and how they would fit in. I was also worried because 10 weeks is a long time. Now two years on and 10 weeks is not long enough!*

Ann gained a great deal of understanding about occupational therapy, its professional mission and philosophy, recognising its similarities with her role within the library context. In this instance of a shared desire to engage older adults in something that is meaningful to them led her to declare:

> *It's been so fantastic I can't wait until next year; it has just been so successful.*
>
> *They have contributed massively. What they do is dedicate five weeks to something we can then take forward. . . . they identified the need for staff training around mental health issues and staff felt able to be open with them about their needs. It's fantastic, that is why we have nominated them for a staff award. They have left us with a legacy.*

The legacy of the student occupational therapists' presence in the library project was multifaceted. The reminiscence project worked well and the original programme design and resources were appreciated by the library staff. Through the students' efforts, some funding was obtained for transportation costs to address the needs of some older adults; the same documentation enabled the on-site supervisor to increase the funding base to provide transportation assistance across the city in a later phase. Creative writing was a focus that had been seen as a priority for some time but had not been established by the time the students started on placement. Ann continues:

> *We couldn't have done it without them . . . I think having these students coming in from the outside, saying nice things about libraries, help staff to understand the important role they play. They also bring the knowledge about the client group which we do not have . . . and knowledge around the importance of engaging with people, essentially that doing things which you enjoy makes you feel better. Their input has been timely with the new personalisation agenda within adult social care whereby day services are closing - a role which libraries may fill in part.*

Despite the obvious value of an occupational therapy view within programmes such as these, Ann doubted that the budget would be allocated to hire occupational therapists within the library system. One of the central value-added components of the role is the natural credibility that comes with it. The supervisor questioned whether librarians would ever be able to enter homes or engage in conversations with clients and be accepted as readily as occurred with the occupational therapy students. This is therefore an area for future focus around establishing a fiscal base for such staffing.

The student perspectives of the 'A Way With Words' project

As earlier, interviews were completed with Kayley and Jasmine which revealed excellent insights concerning the importance of the experience from their perspectives. The student participants commented about the position that libraries held within their communities and the legislated responsibilities identified through their remit as a comprehensive public service responsive to the foci and needs of government initiatives. At the time of placement, a government priority was deemed to be health, and the libraries utilised their commitment to taking an educational approach in meeting these expectations. One student commented:

> *They know they are a traditional service and are keen to evolve, so having a fresh perspective was useful to them. It is difficult when you have been working a certain way for so many years and they are successful. It's just that they want to include more people.*

In the past, this particular library had developed a programme for individuals with mental health issues, but did not meet with much success and the programme closed after only a few sessions from an apparent lack of interest.

> *I don't think they understood the client group and it wasn't really client centred. They had identified mental health as an area of need but unsure how to go about it. I think because it developed out of a librarian's interest in bibliotherapy rather than assessing what people really wanted. It had been a reading group but they hadn't established very strong partnerships, primarily because they didn't know how the NHS worked, whereas we've had experience of working in the NHS.*

Not only did the students' knowledge of the health care system inform and enrich planning for health-based programming, but the specific philosophy and mission of occupational therapy also appeared to have had a particular appeal and relevance.

> *I think introducing the occupational perspective helped them to realise their own value. They were excited about the benefit the libraries could have through the evidence we brought about the benefits of occupational engagement; they were struck by this and we got positive feedback from sharing that. What they were doing it was already there . . . they just need to engage more people.*

Jasmine and Kayley were particularly sensitive to the fact that the library staff had been working in their field for some time, that they had developed strong and helpful services prior to their involvement. The students applied a client-centred, empowering approach with their colleague librarians as well as in their formulation of service programmes for community clients with mental health needs.

> *We made a concerted effort to emphasis how good the service was and that they are experts in their field. It can be a bit daunting if people come in and try to preach to you what you should and shouldn't do. It is a really great service, it's just important that as many people as possible can access it. We did a lot of work around what libraries could offer to people with mental health needs from an occupation perspective, like a sense of routine, sense of well being, and the importance of structure. I don't think they realised that those things could make such a lot of difference.*

Following the collaborative planning between the library staff and the occupational therapy students, the staff reflected that they could see much more clearly approaches they could have used to provide a more relevant service, such as grading activities from outreach visits to the Day Centre, to gradual attendance being established at the library itself. Jasmine and Kayley worked closely with the library staff to articulate the purpose and meaning of activities like creative writing and how critical it is to start from the client's point of departure and not to superimpose interest stemming from the librarians themselves, however well intentioned they may be.

In the past they (the library staff) had probably been more structured and prescriptive whereas we brought the idea of creative freedom in the sessions and gave more options. Our knowledge of the healthcare system and the pathways people go through was helpful and we were familiar with some of the scenarios people found themselves in and able to address them. There was a bit of a culture of fear around mental health. We were a bit shocked at some of the stereotypes that people had. So we were able to break some of those down by talking about our own experiences from past placements. Some didn't know how to communicate with people with mental health needs so that was a learning curve.

One of the students specifically developed a very clear sense of the importance of connecting an occupational perspective with the constructs of community development and social inclusion regarding the role of libraries specifically.

I don't necessarily think it has to be 'OT' unless there was a particular push for 'health through occupation', what is important is how you engage with communities and the value you place on occupation.

Nevertheless the student felt very strongly that the fit with occupational therapy is potentially a very strong one.

Occupational therapists also understand the need for the holistic picture. It's not just about the individual, it's also about assessing the need of the community or group .... I think enabling is a good word ... it's about not doing things for people but empowering them to do it themselves.

Throughout their placement, Jasmine and Kayley utilised evidence from many resources to assist them in forming a picture of the best practice approach with this type of project working with this particular population. Not only did they consult literature and professional colleagues, but also ensured that they were able to gain an understanding of the lived experience from conversing with clients.

An existing creative writing group for 'survivors' of mental health services really guided us. As we were trying to promote participation we wanted to challenge the stigma attached to this group. I think that was one of the things they had got wrong in the past, by labelling their sessions as being for people with mental health needs. Personally that would put me off, so even getting the name of the group was important. We wanted to celebrate participation.

[handwritten margin notes: deprivation to occupational identity due to community ethos support for effective individual occupational status]

Conclusion

The emergence of occupational justice as a conceptual framework necessitates that occupational therapists develop the skills required to work at a macro-level of engagement. The experiences of community development and community psychology professionals can help to inform occupational therapists working in this way. Traditionally, occupational therapy education has focussed upon meeting the needs of individuals; the challenge for occupational therapy educators is to develop population orientated skills in new graduates. These two examples of role emerging placements illustrate how occupational therapy students can bring an occupational perspective to community services and promote community participation and empowerment through occupation. Clearly there is much work still to be done to convince services of the added value which occupational therapists can bring. The students' work highlighted above indicates a clear role in the training and support of frontline staff to deliver meaningful opportunities for engagement and participation with diverse communities. Their skills in assessing occupational need assisted the implementation of projects where previously there had been barriers in their progress, for example, the re-organisation of the physical environment within the initial accommodation site and the emphasis upon client centredness in development of the *A Way with Words* project. Finally these excellent projects are also a credit to the students who undertook them and illustrate their considerable skills and knowledge of the potential power of occupation.

References

Annandale, E. (2003) Socio-economic Inequalities in Health. In Taylor, S. & Field, D. (Eds.), *Sociology of Health and Health Care* 3rd *Edition*. Oxford: Blackwell Publishing, pp. 45–62.

Burnett, A., & Fassil, Y. (2000). *Meeting the health needs of refugee and asylum seekers in the UK: an information and resource pack for health workers*. Department of Health. London: Department of Health.

Burnett, A., & Peel, M. (2001). Health needs of asylum seekers and refugees. *British Medical Journal. 322* (7285), 544–547.

Department for Communities and Local Government's Community Empowerment Division (2006). *Community Development Challenge*. London: Communities and Local Government publications

Freire, P. (1972). *Pedagogy of the Oppressed*. New York: Herder & Herder.

Gower, M. (2009) Asylum seekers and the right to work. London: House of Commons Library, Home Affairs Section. Available from: http://www.parliament.uk/briefingpapers/commons/lib/research/briefings/snha-01908.pdf. [accessed 14/4/10]

Kaseje, D. (1991). Community empowerment, the key to health for all: Keynote address. Paper presented at the Namibian National Network. In: R. Watson & L. Swartz (Eds.), *Transformation through Occupation*. London, Whurr, pp. 57–8.

Kronenberg, F., & Pollard, N. (2005). Overcoming occupational apartheid: a preliminary exploration of the political nature of. In F. Kronenberg, S. S. Algado & N. Pollard (Eds.), *Occupational Therapy Without Borders: Learning from the spirit of survivors*. Oxford: Churchill Livingstone, pp. 58–86

Narayan, D., Patel, R., Schafft, K., Rademacher, A., & Koche-Schulte, S. (2000). *Voices of the poor. Can anyone hear us?* New York: Oxford University Press for the World Bank.

Nelson, G., & Prilleltensky, I. (Eds.). (2005). *Community Psychology. In pursuit of liberation and well-being.* New York: Palgrave MacMillan

Refugee Council Online (2010) Wraparound service. Refugee Council. [Available from: http://www.refugeecouncil.org.uk/howwehelp/directly/main/leeds/Wraparound.htm. [accessed 14/4/10]

Townsend, E., & Wilcock, A. (2003). Occupational Justice. In: Christiansen, C. &. Townsend, E. (Eds.), *Introduction to Occupation. The Art and Science of living.* New Jersey: Prentice Hall, (pp. 243–272).

Tribe, R. (1999). Therapeutic work with refugees living in exile: observations on clinical practice. *Counselling Psychology Quarterly, 12* (3), 233–243.

Watson, R. (2004). New horizons in occupational therapy, In; Watson, R., & Swartz, L. (2004). *Transformation through occupation.* London: Wiley. (pp. 3–18)

Whiteford, E. (2004). When people cannot participate: Occupational deprivation. In: C. Townsend (Ed.), *Introduction to Occupation. The Art and Science of Living.* New Jersey: Prentice Hall, (pp. 221–242).

United Nations. (1951). *Convention and Protocol Relating to the Status of Refugees.* Geneva: UNHCR.

Whiteford, G., Townsend, E., & Hocking, C. (2000). Reflections on a Renaissance of Occupation. *Canadian Journal of Occupational Therapy, 67* (1), 61-69.

Wilcock, A. (1998). *An Occupational Perspective of Health.* Thorofare, NJ: Slack.

Yerxa, E. J. (1998). Occupation: The keystone of a curriculum for a self-defined profession. *The American Journal of Occupational Therapy : Official Publication of the American Occupational Therapy Association. 52* (5), 365–372.

Part III

Future of the profession

We are now at the point in the book where many readers may be asking themselves "Now what?" The importance of appreciating our past has been introduced as a good place to start in envisioning our future; the importance of embracing a congruent and connected view of academic preparation of students and the practice experiences that help them to be grounded and to apply the theoretical learning to real life dilemmas and tragedies has been detailed.

We have been given the opportunity to join learners, faculty and community preceptors in their descriptions of many diverse emerging practice experiences. Perhaps, through reading about these examples of non-traditional fieldwork, we have been inspired to think differently and perhaps something has triggered an idea that has been lying dormant or not even recognised until now.

Many chapter authors have detailed fieldwork experiences that have arisen from unique opportunities outside the usual institutional and community settings, working with client groups that do not necessarily become identified by a diagnosis, but rather from the issues and problems they face. This would seem to be a very obvious invitation for occupational therapists to step up to the plate and declare our unique contribution to the endeavour of living 'well'; that is, attention to 'occupation' as the central construct and one which can apply to anyone at any time in life. These examples have explored the 'fit' between the person and the occupation with much attention to the environment.

The final section of this book will address issues related to the importance of systemic innovation through attention to policy changes opening doors to innovative practice models. The future of our profession will be discussed with a view to 'pushing the envelope' and embracing what can be perhaps the richest chapter in our history yet.

Chapter 10

Using policy and government drivers to create role emerging opportunities

Lori Letts & Julie Richardson

Introduction

Role emerging clinical placement opportunities can be identified through a number of strategies. One promising area is to consider transitions in health and social policies and service delivery to guide the identification and development of such placements for students. In this chapter, a number of research and policy transitions are presented that may guide considerations and lead to opportunities for role emerging placements. These were used by investigators of the Community Scholar project to guide their work. Details of the Community Scholar project are shared here, and lessons learned from the initiative are described.

Policy transitions

Over recent decades, influences within broad health policy and transitions in health care (including occupational therapy) practice have increased the attention paid to public and community health. Emphasis has been placed on the importance of inter-professional collaboration in both delivery and education of health care providers. Key transitions in policy and practice have included a focus on public health, and within that the determinants of health, health promotion and disease/disability prevention, as well as emphasis on renewal in primary health care.

Public health

Nutbeam (1998, p. 3) defined public health as "a social and political concept aimed at improving health, prolonging life and improving the quality of life among whole populations through health promotion, disease prevention and other forms of health intervention". Public health as a concept and policy driver has been in place for decades, yet more recently it has received more attention in health policy. Key aspects of public health policies have included increased emphasis on the determinants of health, health promotion and community or population health.

Role Emerging Occupational Therapy: Maximising Occupation-Focused Practice, 1st edition. Edited by Miranda Thew, Mary Edwards, Sue Baptiste and Matthew Molineux. © 2011 Blackwell Publishing Ltd.

Determinants of health

As health has come to be understood as more than the absence of disease, a broader definition of health has led to more holistic understandings of the factors that influence and affect health. Broadly known as the determinants of health, these are the multiple and multifaceted factors that influence people's feelings of health and well-being. The Public Health Agency of Canada (2001a, ¶ 3) notes that "at every stage of life, health is determined by complex interactions between social and economic factors, the physical environment and individual behavior" which are known as the determinants of health. The determinants of health are described in various ways, but typically include income and socio-economic status, gender, social supports, physical and social environments, cultural environments, education, working conditions, health services, genetic factors and personal health practices (Letts, 2009; Public Health Agency of Canada, 2001a). With determinants of health as a focus of health policy development, a number of strategies have emerged including disease prevention and health promotion, both of which have a focus on addressing broad determinants of health as strategies to improve health and prevent disease, rather than responding to and treating health conditions as they occur.

Health promotion

Health promotion is most frequently defined as a "process of enabling people to increase control over and improve their health" (World Health Organization, 1986, p. 2). Some of the main tenants of health promotion include: community participation, empowerment, social justice, greater autonomy for the community, the importance of active and meaningful lifestyles, and respect for cultural diversity (Thibeault & Hebert, 1997).

Community health

With influences from public health, the determinants of health, health promotion and prevention, policy tends to focus at the levels of groups, communities and entire populations, rather than solely addressing health issues for individuals. There has been a transition to refocus from individuals to communities and populations (Gahimer & Morris, 1999). At national levels, governments frequently set health targets or goals for the population. For example, in Canada, Ministers of Health at the national, provincial and territorial levels agreed on the Health Goals for Canada in October 2005 (Public Health Agency of Canada, 2009). Population health has become an important policy context, in that the goal of population health is "an approach to health that aims to improve the health of the entire population and to reduce health inequities among population groups" (Public Health Agency of Canada, 2001b, ¶ 1).

Population health frequently relies on epidemiological data at population levels. Through such national health data sets as the Canadian Community Health Survey, increasing attention has been paid to the determinants of health and the increasing prevalence of chronic diseases. A need has been identified to help address the needs of people with chronic diseases, to optimise their health and prevent disabling conditions. Therefore, an emphasis on improving community health services has resulted, which has included the recognition of the need to address community health through reforms in the primary health care system, including improved approaches to chronic disease management, and increased inter-professional collaboration and education to better prepare health professionals to work in the newly reformed health system.

Primary health care reform

In countries such as the United Kingdom (UK) and Canada, reform of the system of providing primary health care has been underway over the past two decades. This has included attention to both the ways in which primary health care services have been provided and funded. In Canada, primary care reform has been led through the creation of a primary health care transition fund (started in 2000), a first ministers' health accord in 2003 with a focus on increasing the access to primary care services for more Canadians, and in 2004 with the development of new targets to meet the goals of the 2003 accord (Health Canada, 2004). In the UK, primary care reform has been initiated for a number of reasons including the aging population, the increased ease with which complex conditions are managed in community settings and the increasing prevalence of chronic diseases (Schoen et al., 2009). This reform is described in one document as comprising four directions: practice-based commissioning, shifting resources into prevention, encouraging innovation and allowing different providers to compete for services (Department of Health, 2006). Kerr and Scott (2009) suggest that the strength of health reforms undertaken in the UK can be attributed to the successes in primary health care reform.

Primary care reform seems driven by a number of factors, and has included efforts to address not only the ways in which services are provided, but the need to focus on addressing the needs of people with chronic illnesses, and delivery of services in a way that best addresses those needs, including the provision of inter-professional services within community settings (Health Council of Canada, 2007).

Inter-professional collaboration and education

Inter-professional collaboration is a thread noted in relation to community health, primary health care and chronic disease management. Teams composed of many disciplines or professions are seen as the ideal way in which improved population health can be achieved. In Canada, the Primary Health Care Transition Fund supported a pan-Canadian initiative that focused on reforming primary health care to increase inter-professional collaborations in optimising health outcomes for Canadians (Enhancing Interdisciplinary Collaboration in Primary Health Care, 2006). For inter-professional collaboration to be successful in health care, health professionals need to learn more about one another and how best to work together (Headrick et al., 1998). Inter-professional education (IPE) is defined as occasions when "two or more professions learn with, from and about each other to improve collaboration and the quality of care" (Centre for the Advancement of Inter-professional Education, 2002). Although there are many approaches to IPE, Barr (2007) described three foci of IPE initiatives: "preparing individuals for collaborative practice; learning to work in teams; developing services to improve care" (p. 40); and added a fourth: improving quality of life in communities. In his description of the fourth foci, Barr highlighted a number of strategies in which IPE initiatives could be directed, including offering students opportunities to learn about community health issues, and placing students in community health placements. The project described in this chapter built on many of the policy transitions described above to create an inter-professional education opportunity designed to address the fourth focus of IPE described by Barr.

Case example: the Community Scholar Project

The Community Scholar Project emerged as a means of linking academic curricula content in community health to clinical practice. At McMaster University, many of the health professional education programmes had already made shifts to reflect these transitions (e.g. Richardson & Letts, 2005). The project offered an opportunity for students to gain skills and knowledge in community health, and to do so through inter-professional education. The intent of the project was for students from occupational therapy, physiotherapy, nursing and medical programmes to interact with one another and with other members of health and social-service teams. The stimulus for the project was in large part the fact that academic curricula in the health professional programmes included content related to health policy transitions and community health, but there were few student placement opportunities for students to understand or apply the skills and knowledge they were gaining in the academic programmes. The project process and outcomes from the perspective of students and preceptors are described in detail in a paper by Richardson et al. (2009).

The main goal of the project was to design, implement and evaluate a training programme for an inter-professional community scholar. Community scholars referred to the students involved in the initiatives associated with the project. The project had two main threads of learning for the students participating as community scholars. The first thread was community health and the second was inter-professional education. These were addressed through three main activities: inter-professional clinical fieldwork experiences, connections with community leaders, and mentorship. The project is described in more detail in Richardson et al. (2009), including a programme logic model. Throughout all three of the main activities in which the students participated, it was anticipated that they would gain knowledge about community health issues; they would come to have increased knowledge and skill about how their own discipline could address those community health issues, while simultaneously gaining knowledge about how other disciplines might address the same issues. Because they were learning together and working in inter-professional contexts, it was anticipated that the students would gain knowledge and skills in inter-professional practice.

In terms of the practice placement education experiences, four sites hosted students, whereas other partners provided opportunities for meetings with community leaders. The four sites included:

- Hamilton YWCA
- McMaster Family Health Team (with students at two sites: Stonechurch Family Health Centre and McMaster Family Practice)
- Shelter Health Network.

Each of the sites that agreed to take students offered opportunities for learning in relation to the communities they served. All but the YWCA had access to medical and nursing services for their clients; none of the sites had provided physiotherapy or occupational therapy service in the past. The YWCA is primarily a membership-based organisation. The students were involved in different programmes offered, including fitness programmes for people with specific conditions (e.g. BoneBuilders for people with osteoarthritis, HeartBeat for people with cardiac conditions) as well as programmes offered for older adults living independently in the community. The McMaster Family Health Team is comprised of two primary health care sites offering inter-professional primary health care to patients. Academic family physicians at the sites hold faculty appointments in the Department of Family Medicine at McMaster University, and practice with community physicians and inter-professional team members in two major teaching units: Stonechurch Family Health Centre and McMaster Family Practice. The Shelter Health Network (www.shelterhealthnetwork.ca) provides primary health care and other support services to shelter residents in the city of Hamilton. Shelter users are a heterogeneous group of persons who are without housing or in transitional housing and include a mobile population of single men, women, families, youth, visible minorities and aboriginal people many who have serious physical and mental health problems. Typically, health services are provided by a combination of family physicians, nurse practitioners, nurses, social workers, psychiatrists and others.

At each of the sites, student placements were supported through the allocation of space and instrumental supports to orient the students to the site, creating interaction opportunities with clients/patients served at the sites, offering opportunities for the students to learn about community health issues from the perspectives of the organisations and the people they served.

The second activity of the experience linked students with community leaders who discussed the health issues facing people within the Hamilton community. Students made linkages with staff and clients of the Hostel to Home project and accessed a multidisciplinary course in Poverty and Homelessness, and met with representatives from the Hamilton Community Foundation, the City of Hamilton Public Health and Community Services Department. The third activity involved the faculty members and project investigators mentoring students as they presented cases and discussed the issues in relation to community health and inter-professional collaboration. The mentorship was an opportunity for students to learn from and with each other, with support of faculty members to integrate some of their experiences and consider how they contributed to the students' emerging understandings of community health and inter-professional practice.

In planning the evaluation of this project, a number of stakeholders were identified who would be able to provide input into the evaluation of the project. These included students, preceptors/supervisors, community agencies hosting students on placement, community leaders meeting with students, mentors and clients/patients of the programmes with which students were involved. Of these six groups, a decision was made to focus the evaluation on five groups of stakeholders (students, preceptors, community agencies, mentors and community leaders). Although the long-term goal of the project was to improve the health of the community members receiving service through the community agencies, we did not include the service recipients in the evaluation for two main reasons. First, in planning the project, it was very difficult to know how or how many clients the students would work with through their placements. Without a clear idea of the ways in which the students would connect with clients, it was impossible to plan for a process to include clients in the evaluation, in light of the need for review and approval by the Research Ethics Board. Further, many of the agencies work with clients/patients who are in marginalised groups, who may have already been burdened through their circumstance. Since the focus of the evaluation was primarily on the processes involved in integrating the students into the environments, it seemed most appropriate to concentrate on organisational and learner stakeholders. However, community agencies were asked to provide feedback on whether clients of their agencies benefited from the students' presence, providing some input on at least their perception of the benefits offered to clients through the project.

Evaluation

Five stakeholder groups were engaged in the evaluation. Data from the students was gathered through three mechanisms. First, students collected data on a reflective journal that was specifically designed for the project (Box 10.1). As well, students tracked their inter-professional experiences at three levels: exposure, immersion and mastery. These levels are described by McMaster University's Programme for Inter-professional Practice, Education and Research (PIPER; 2010). Students were expected to participate in at least one activity under each of the three levels by the end of their involvement in the project. Finally, at the end of each placement education experience, students participated with the investigators in a focus group to discuss their experiences with the project, and to provide input on their learning in relation to community health and inter-professional practice.

  Preceptors evaluated the experiences by participating in a focus group at the end of each placement block. In total, three focus groups were held with preceptors. Representatives

---

Box 10.1   Reflective journal template

Incident: Describe the basics of what occurred – date, who was involved, some detail about what happened.
Communication: Reflect on how the incident is linked to communication with others at the site or who were involved in the interaction; this might include other students, preceptors, patients/clients or team members at the site.
Community health: Reflect on how the incident links to your understandings of community health issues at the specific site or more generally.
Inter-professional practice issues: Reflect on how the incident is linked to your understandings of other health professions. What new insights have you gained about the contributions of other professionals to community health? What questions do you have about other health professions?
Profession-specific practice issues: Reflect on how the incident is linked to your own development as a health professional and within your discipline. For example, what is the role of your profession in this setting? What are the possibilities that you see? Do others see them? How is the role different from what you learned in school?

from the community agencies and the community leaders evaluated the experience by responding to an on-line survey conducted immediately after the first two rounds of placements. The surveys focused on the benefits and challenges to the agencies, their clients, and the students through their interactions. They were asked to describe the types of interactions they had with the students. Community agencies hosting the sites were also asked if they would be willing to host students again in future.

Results

The project was implemented in three rounds for six-week student placements at the participating community sites. Recruitment of students and their participation in placements at the various sites are summarised in Table 10.1. Recruitment of occupational therapy and physiotherapy students was easier than that from nursing and medicine. Nonetheless, there were two times when either an OT or a PT student was placed without a fellow student from another discipline. In these situations, efforts were undertaken to integrate students from similar sites and other disciplines, and also to maximise opportunities for these students to interact with other members of the health care team to maximise inter-professional learning. The challenges experienced in recruiting nursing and medical students to the project in the first two rounds included difficulties with timing in the curricula (e.g. nursing students were placed for longer periods but fewer hours each week), and limited abilities to locate preceptors to supervise students. As such, for the third round of placements, students were placed at only two sites and an embedded recruitment approach was used, which meant recruiting learners from nursing and medicine who were already participating in on-site placement experiences with a preceptor assigned.

Table 10.1 Summary of student placements by site and round.

Site	Round 1	Round 2	Round 3
Shelter Health Network	OT/PT	OT/PT	
YWCA	OT/PT	OT/PT	
Stonechurch Health Centre	OT	OT/PT	OT/PT/Nurse practitioner/ medical residents
McMaster Family Practice	OT/PT	OT/PT	OT/PT/medical residents

Feedback from students and preceptors

Students enrolled in the community scholar project gained significant new understandings of inter-professional collaboration and community health through involvement in the project. Results from the focus groups with students (summarised by Richardson et al., 2009) suggest that the opportunities for learning together and positive interactions with one another and the team were important contributions to their learning related to inter-professional collaboration. Students had opportunities to collaborate on providing direct service to clients and also to prepare education seminars to staff and clients at the sites. In terms of community health, they gained new learning about community resources and each site offered them unique learning opportunities. Preceptors reported the experience of the community scholar as positive for the students they supervised as well as for themselves. They reported significant support for the types of placements that offered opportunities for students to learn about community health issues, community resources and determinants of health. They reported some challenges in working to support students when they were supervising the students in agencies with which they were not familiar, but reported managing this by facilitating the students in their understandings of how the agencies worked. They noted that students placed together worked well and had significant inter-professional education experiences, both with one another and with other members of the team.

Feedback from mentors

All mentors agreed that the mentorship meetings supported students in their learning about community health and inter-professional education. They offered students broad exposure to community health issues; by bringing together learners from different sites, students were exposed to a broader range of issues faced in different settings. Discussions during the meetings highlighted diversity in issues but also the importance of the determinants of health, community resources and IPE across a variety of situations. All agreed that informal mentorship meetings met students' learning needs, while creating a comfortable and safe learning environment. The inter-professional nature of the meetings also meant that students could learn with and from other disciplines, thus supporting IPE.

Feedback from community agencies

Through the responses to on-line surveys with representatives from agencies that hosted students on placement, there was unanimous support for the initiative. All respondents ($n = 14$) agreed that the partnership with McMaster through the community scholar project should continue. Respondents were also unanimous that students were adequately prepared for the placement. Thirteen respondents agreed that clients of the agencies benefited from having students at the agency, and the respondent who replied 'no' clarified the no meant "not sure, I really have not heard back from any clients on their experience except a few who said they were assessed and then nothing happened". When asked to describe the ways in which students assisted clients, responses included: "They were able to ask more in depth questions about their health and functional living challenges that they face on a day to day basis. Questions that were beyond the scope of the staff", and "Our clients benefited enormously, there is no doubt in my mind that many of them would not have gained access to these services had it not been for the students".

Feedback from community leaders

Community leaders were members of the broader community who met with students for one or two occasions to support students' learning related to community health issues.

Responses from the community leaders about their interactions with the students were generally positive, highlighting the opportunity the interactions allowed them to provide the students with insights into community health issues for the population served by their organisations. Although most felt that students benefited from the interactions, only one third reported learning something new from the students. All agreed that the students benefited from learning gained from their interactions.

Discussion

There were some consistent challenges and supports identified through the evaluation across stakeholder groups. There was unanimous support from students, preceptors, mentors, agencies and community leaders that students gained new understandings of community health issues, the contributions their own disciplines could make and the nature of inter-professional collaborations to promote health with diverse communities. At each of the four placement sites, significant time and energy went into the development of the sites. This involved collaboration and frequent communication between the university investigators and the partner sites. An agency contact was designated to be a support to the students, to provide orientation and regular input to make sure the students were integrated to the sites. These contact people provided immense support for the students and preceptors in their integration in each of the sites. Over the course of the three rounds of student placements, the students developed resource materials to forward to the next group, so that each student group entering a site benefited from materials, resources and suggestions from the last set of students. In this way, despite new learners entering the site for each round, an effort was made to 'pass on' the learning gained from previous students.

Although three of the four sites provided medical and nursing services, none of them provided rehabilitation to their clients with any consistency. The presence of the community scholar students provided sites with an opportunity to see and understand the contributions that rehabilitation could make to promote health with clients served by the sites.

The project did encounter some challenges. At all four sites, space for students to provide services to clients was limited. Students did not always have consistent access to assessment or treatment spaces to see clients; nor did they have consistent access to office space, or communication equipment at all sites. Equipment sometimes had to be borrowed or purchased for the students to provide services. For example, the students at all sites except one had access to a hi-lo bed to see clients for assessment and intervention. At the site where this was not available, students were sometimes challenged in how best to conduct a physical rehabilitation assessment with clients. At sites that were community or social-services agencies, there were challenges for the students to maintain and store health records; the students, preceptors and investigators worked together to ensure a system was established that followed regulatory agency standards for documentation. At all four sites, systems needed to be developed to enable referrals and to support communications between students, team members and clients served by the organisations.

Recruiting students for simultaneous learning opportunities from four disciplines proved difficult to coordinate. This resulted from variations in curricula organisation and timing. Although the embedded approach used in the third round offered improved IPE opportunities, it continued to be challenging. Nonetheless, linking students with professionals from each community agency resulted in rich inter-professional learning, even though not all of the people involved were learners or at the same level of learning.

Several factors will determine the sustainability of this project. First, it is important for educational and administrative leaders from partner organisations to support the initiative. Although there is support in principle from all partners to continue the partnership, financial resources need to be acquired to continue with the Community Scholar initiative. Optimally, if the experiences developed for this project are sustained, they will become routine inter-professional collaborations. The main barrier to sustainability is the lack of ongoing funding for the preceptors to supervise students. This is true for rehabilitation students at all sites, and also for nursing and medical students if they were to be placed at agencies such as the YWCA in which those disciplines do not have a professional presence.

Applying the lessons learned

The Community Scholar Project has illustrated how an inter-professional collaborative project based in community–university partnerships can take advantage of policy transitions. In this case, our project relied heavily on a trend towards inter-professional collaboration to fund an initiative with a focus on community health, determinants of health and health promotion. Three main lessons might be helpful in the development of future role emerging placements grounded in policy transitions such as this one:

i) Partnerships take significant time and effort from both sides. By placing students in sites where rehabilitation professionals had no presence, the sites, university programmes, preceptors and students were all challenged to create the infrastructure to support the students to learn while providing useful services to clients and staff within the organisations. Important aspects of infrastructure included allocating space and equipment for the students to be able to work within the agencies. Consistent and frequent communications were needed to ensure that referrals, documentation and resources were organised. We were able to build these components over time, and improve the efficiency of the systems; however, each organisation was unique and required nuanced understanding.

ii) Through the project, we have come to believe that it is important for students to select the initiative or site for their learning. Students were presented with many challenges during their role emerging placements. They worked with clients who often faced significant health and social challenges; some were homeless or had very tenuous housing. Some had very complex health and living situations, resulting in the students feeling at times as if they had little to offer the clients. Some settings required more of a health education or promotion emphasis from students, which challenged them when they were more interested in providing health or rehabilitation services using more traditional models of service delivery. Through observations, reviewing student reflective journals and discussions in the focus groups, it became clear that learning for students was very challenging and was in part facilitated because they had been involved in choosing the site for their placements.

iii) We have concluded that preceptors need to be strong clinicians, often generalists, with willingness to take on new learning themselves. All of the preceptors were required to demonstrate tremendous flexibility in supporting student learning; at times they were involved in supporting students from other health professions. Although they expressed some concerns that they were frustrated not to have the kind of 'insider' information they would typically have when supervising students in their own organisations, they demonstrated an ability to help the students gain access and information needed to support their learning.

Conclusions

Students enrolled in the community scholar project gained significant new understandings of inter-professional collaboration and community health through involvement in the project. Our results suggest that the opportunities for learning together and positive interactions with one another and the team were important contributions to their learning related to inter-professional collaboration. Students had opportunities to collaborate on providing direct service to clients, and also to prepare education seminars to staff and clients at the sites. In terms of community health, they gained new learning about community resources and each site offered them unique learning opportunities. The community scholar project was built on a premise that academic curricula influenced by policy transitions can be supported through the development of role emerging placements that translate academic curricula into practice. As health policies continue to evolve, lessons from the project could be applied in developing new role emerging placements for students in a variety of health profession programmes, including student occupational therapists.

References

Barr, H. (2007). Inter-professional education: the fourth focus. *Journal of Inter-professional Care*, *21*(Suppl. 2), 40–50.

Centre for the Advancement of Inter-professional Education (CAIPE). (2002). Defining IPE. Retrieved November 27, 2009 from http://www.caipe.org.uk/about-us/defining-ipe/.

Department of Health. (2006). *Our health our care our say: A new direction for community services. Retrieved from:* http://www.dh.gov.uk/en/Publicationsandstatistics/Publications/PublicationsPolicyAndGuidance/Browsable/DH_4127552.

Enhancing Interdisciplinary Collaboration in Primary Health Care. (2006). *Primary health care: A framework that fits*. Retrieved from http://www.eicp.ca/en/.

Gahimer, J. E., & Morris, D. M. (1999). Community health education: Evolving opportunities for physical therapists. *Journal of Physical Therapy Education*, *13* (3), 38–48.

Health Canada. (2004). Primary health care and health system renewal (updated 2004-10-01). Retrieved January 1, 2010 from http://www.hc-sc.gc.ca/hcs-sss/prim/renew-renouv-eng.php.

Health Council of Canada. (2007). *Why health care renewal matters: Learning from Canadians with chronic health conditions*. Ottawa, ON: Author.

Headrick, L. A., Wilcock, P. M., & Batalden, P. B. (1998). Inter-professional working and continuing medical education. *British Medical Journal, 316*, 771-774. Retrieved from: http://www.bmj.com.libaccess.lib.mcmaster.ca/cgi/content/full/316/7133/771.

Improving Chronic Illness Care. (n.d.). *The Chronic Care Model Gallery.* Retrieved from http://www.improvingchroniccare.org/index.php?p=CCM_Gallery&s=149.

Kerr, D. J., & Scott, M. (2009). British lessons on health care reform. *New England Journal of Medicine, Volume 361:e21* (13). DOI: 10.1056/NEJMp0906618.

Letts, L. (2009). Health promotion. In E. B. Crepeau, E. Cohn, & B. A. B. Schell (Eds.), *Willard & Spackman's Occupational Therapy* (11th ed., pp. 165–180). Baltimore: Wolters Kluwer Lippincott, Williams & Wilkins.

Nutbeam, D. (1998). *Health promotion glossary.* Geneva: World Health Organization. Retrieved 22 July 2005, from http://whqlibdoc.who.int/hq/1998/WHO_HPR_HEP_98.1.pdf.

Programme for Inter-professional Practice, Education and Research (PIPER). (2010). Competencies and levels: Description of IPE activities and competencies. Retrieved from: http://piper.mcmaster.ca/about_competencies.html.

Public Health Agency of Canada. (2001a). *What determines health?* (updated 2001-12-08). Retrieved 27 November 2009 from http://www.phac-aspc.gc.ca/ph-sp/determinants/index-eng.php#determinants.

Public Health Agency of Canada. (2001b). *What is the population health approach?* (updated 2001-12-08). Retrieved 1 January 2010 from http://www.phac-aspc.gc.ca/ph-sp/approach-approche/index-eng.php.

Public Health Agency of Canada. (2009). *Health goals for Canada* (updated 2009-12-01). Retrieved 1 December 2009 from http://www.phac-aspc.gc.ca/hgc-osc/home.html.

Richardson, J., & Letts, L. (2005). Curricula to promote community health. In P. Solomon & S. Baptiste (Eds.), *Problem-based learning in rehabilitation* (pp. 113–133). Berlin, Germany: Springer-Verlag.

Richardson, J., Letts, L., Childs, A., Semogas, D., Stavness, C., Smith, B. J., Guenter, D., & Price, D. (2009). Development of a community scholar programme: An inter-professional initiative. *Journal of Physical Therapy Education, 24*, 39–45.

Schoen, C., Osborn, R., Doty, M. M., Squires, D., Peugh, J., & Applebaum, S. (2009). A survey of primary care physicians in eleven countries, 2009: Perspectives on care, costs and experiences. *Health Affairs, 28* (6), w1171–w1183. doi: 10.1377/hlthaff.28.6.w1171

Thibeault, R., & Hebert, M. (1997). A congruent model for health promotion in occupational therapy. *Occupational Therapy International, 4*, 271–293.

World Health Organization. (1986). *Ottawa charter for health promotion: 1st International conference on health promotion:.* Geneva: Author. Retrieved from http://www.who.int/healthpromotion/conferences/previous/ottawa/en/print.html

Chapter 11

The way forward?

Sue Baptiste & Matthew Molineux

Introduction

This chapter will reflect upon the accomplishments and stories of the contributors to the preceding chapters and the work in which they have engaged against a backdrop of past, present and developing foci and scope of occupational therapy practice. The examples illustrated within this book provide some sense of the scope of future occupational therapy roles and professional contributions to the health and well-being of the people of the world. These are some of the new steps being taken in the developing journey of the profession. Many changes can be seen in the ways we, as practitioners, engage with clients and embrace responsibilities within the populations with whom we work. This book focuses particularly upon some of the bright and innovative opportunities for our students in their fieldwork experiences, thus preparing practitioners with an open approach to practice possibilities. Trends for the new century, and potentially beyond, will be explored and thoughts from the authors shared concerning the reframing of societal needs in relation to occupation and health.

The context of the past and present

As stated in Chapter 1, in little more than a century the profession of occupational therapy has laid down roots based on historical patterns, developed core roles and practice expectations, dealt with identity struggles and emerged with a developing and unique body of knowledge and skills (Friedland, 2003; Townsend & Polatajko, 2007). A new science of occupation has also arisen from this intense inquiry into the essence of our work and has provided us with a new lens to view our practice and profession. Engaging in research and using evidence to support best practices are becoming more the norm than the exception, to the point that the field of occupational science has carved a strong foothold beyond the boundaries of applied practice. This has encouraged the development of partnerships with other academic disciplines in exploring ideas and concepts related to occupation more broadly.

Role Emerging Occupational Therapy: Maximising Occupation-Focused Practice, 1st edition. Edited by Miranda Thew, Mary Edwards, Sue Baptiste and Matthew Molineux. © 2011 Blackwell Publishing Ltd.

Occupational therapy as a profession grew from a place of 'doing' as many skilled historians have detailed (Wilcock, 1998; Friedland, 2003). Initial roles were created and played out in rehabilitation units, hospital settings and post-war (World Wars I and II) environments. The growth of the profession itself was realised in parallel with the practice scope, from physical rehabilitation to mental health and work/productivity re-entry. It was the practical nature of the discipline that was the focus for several decades with major attention being paid to the provision of practice experiences as a critical component of the core of the professional preparation and training programmes (Friedland, 2003).

Community involvement naturally became a practice component as people were discharged home from institutions or into care facilities, yet still requiring follow-up treatment, maintenance and monitoring. However, earlier practice models were predicated on the expectation that institutionally based staff members would provide the home service for relatively brief periods of time. As a result, rehabilitation continued to be located in institutions. Slowly the need for community-based services became clear and then a fracture between the institution and society began to emerge. Independent services were creating a challenge to the continuance of the original flow of care (Kielhofner, 2004).

The professional frame of reference and supportive model of practice remained that of the medical model, as illustrated in Chapter 1, to the point that, in the 1970s occupational therapists tended to become 'mini-everything' – physiotherapists, counsellors, recreation therapists, nursing affiliates in long-term care and psychotherapists in community psychiatry (Gottesfeld et al., 1970; Jacoby & Oppenheimer, 1991; Sayce et al., 1991; Finlay, 1993). Occupational therapists were floundering in their attempts to understand and enact their unique contributions to the health care delivery enterprise. It was then that radical changes began to occur. Despite the relatively languid pace at which these changes were wrought, the overall pace of professional evolution gathered speed from that time to the present. We would seem to be poised now on the cusp of even more dramatic innovations appearing from the reorganisation and restructuring of health care systems and social agencies; often enabled through the enactment of emerging fieldwork experiences that, in themselves, will enable an exciting growth within the profession as a whole (Brown & Rodger, 2006; Canadian Association of Occupational Therapists, 2007).

The profession's commitment to certain foundational practice models became rooted in the inter-relationships between individuals, the occupations in which they engage and the environments within which those occupations are undertaken. A strong commitment to the central construct of 'occupation' emerged, at the (perhaps rightful) expense of attachment to the medical frame of reference. The development of a unique body of knowledge was seen to be a priority (Law et al., 1993; Mathiowetz, 1993) as well as the creation of outcome measures that would address occupation rather than physical, cognitive and affective elements in the context of 'function' and 'activity' (Carswell et al, 2004). Theoretical frameworks were created as the top level of a taxonomy of theory, and then linked to existing knowledge in the biological and social sciences. Questions were asked about the wisdom of remaining linked only to rehabilitation. Other partnerships were explored and formed with colleagues in disciplines such as social work, geography, epidemiology, public health and government and policy (e.g. Leathard, 2003). Research and inquiry related to occupation were pursued with passion and animation. As referred to in Chapter 1, the growth of occupational science provided an ideal environment in which to nurture collaborative and broad-reaching academic relationships. A business approach to occupational therapy practice has also gained traction over the last two decades in particular since more and more practitioners have taken the path to private practice, thus requiring different skill sets such as marketing, business plan development, the writing of programme proposals and funding applications, as well as the centrality of advocacy – with consumers to government and other funders/supporters/resources as well as for the profession itself.

Grasping contemporary opportunity to guide the future

When we agreed to collaborate to develop this book, we all came to the realisation that it seemed timely for reasons that we held in common from The United Kingdom to Australia to Canada. This was a very powerful recognition for us; the sense of common purpose and experience was upheld in finding authors who would share experiments and innovations that illustrate our mutual insights, and also to reflect on differences and commonalities across cultural and geographic boundaries.

Emerging trends

Primary health care

For many years, there have been major efforts expended within the health care system in Canada, and indeed elsewhere, to establish a place for occupational therapy within the primary health care environment. Most recently in Canada, occupational therapy has become an accepted and expected member of the primary health care team within community doctors' offices and family health teams (Ministry of Health & Long Term Care Ontario, 2010). Such efforts and roles have been well expounded in Chapter 10, in which Letts and Richardson offer their experiences within primary health and in particular, with self-management of chronic disease strategies offered as a prime model for showing the value of rehabilitation disciplines at the front line. Establishing ourselves within this critical component of health care services would seem eminently sensible.

Working with diagnosis-free populations

Our allegiance has shifted from seeing the medical model as the only one that fits our contributions, and thus there is no need to stay hooked into a view that constructs our clients from the perspective of impairment, illness, diagnosis and disability. The World Health Organization (2010) has played a key part in changing how population data are viewed around the globe with the development of the International Classification of Function, which is the latest iteration of the original International Classification of Illness, Disease and Handicap. The new model has adopted a language consistent with occupation by creating a new framework around the constructs of illness, activity and participation. Not only are we supported in our client-centred approach by this model but we are led towards seeing our work as detached from diagnoses and framed instead by issues of occupational engagement that are central to each potential client's participation in his world.

However, linking our work to diagnostically identified client populations can present opportunities to address matters of occupational engagement instead of staying focused at the impairment level. Brown and Gurney (Chapter 8) speak of the development of an occupational therapy presence within a community clinic for people experiencing cardiac failure. This is not a traditional role by any means, yet this unfolds as a sensible and valuable application of occupational therapy knowledge and skills.

There is nothing to say that occupational therapists should ignore the notion of working with 'well' people in times of crisis or transition in their lives as noted in Chapter 1 in relation to the Well Elderly Study (Clark et al, 1997). There are the more obvious opportunities within various programmes aimed at prevention (e.g. work injuries, falls). Both Thew and Hall (Chapters 5 and 6 respectively), in their different but equally informative and innovative accounts of their roles within established organisations, take different approaches to what has been a well recognised role for occupational therapy. Other roles that can become a good 'fit' for the application of occupational therapy involve perhaps working as a catalyst, facilitator and/or advocate with and for community groups needing such guidance and support. Potential client groups could include groups of older adults looking for assistance and support in planning retirement, reinforcing learned skills and maximising their worth to their communities. Other examples may well spring to mind such as partnering with young adults with disabilities as they make the leap from childhood and adolescence to adulthood; in this context, these young people are well and are not considering their disability as an illness or condition to take priority in their decision-making.

Community front-line settings working with marginalised populations

Trentham and Cockburn (Chapter 7) provide a clear vision for working with community health centres and establishing a niche by partnering with individuals living with longstanding mental illness and other chronic problems; these people often represent a cross-section of a large urban community. Building on the community health centre model, there are more and more opportunities for engaging with immigrant and refugee programmes, as outlined and highlighted within this text. The importance of occupational engagement for transient or relocating populations cannot be overemphasised. Critical connections need to be established and supported in order to enable new citizens in their search for integration and acculturation to the context and culture of their new home.

Windley (Chapter 9) speaks to the notion of students working within a refugee centre and a community-based library with a programme for clients with mental health concerns. In both of these placement sites, the students speak of feeling that they have made a difference and that they have carved out new ground for the application of concepts related to health and occupation. The support of on-site supervisors not from an occupational therapy background is identified as a central success indicator. This in itself provides a clear link back to the discussions around models of and planning for successful role emerging placements as offered by Edwards and Thew (Chapter 2) and Roger and Thomas (Chapter 3).

Public education

On a temporary basis, many occupational therapists have undertaken public education endeavours within public spaces such as shopping malls and special community celebrations. Although these are short-lived examples of changing our professional focus, they can also be integral components of emerging role placements. In addition, this approach could be embellished and enriched through a commitment to working with other health professionals and social-service agencies in providing a client-centred approach towards single parents and their children, newly bereaved middle-aged and older adults as well as street youth and the homeless. The professional literature is becoming well populated with examples of occupational therapists breaking new ground and becoming involved and invested in working with such potentially marginalised populations. The needs of prison inmates remain an area not well explored by occupational therapists but are a dramatic example of occupational deprivation (Whiteford, 2000). There may well be rich opportunities to work with inmates approaching parole and facing re-entry into their communities including family, work and social context. In addition, preparation with new coping skills could bode well for a better-organised life that will steer away from previously destructive habits. There will be a central need for practitioners to become comfortable with developing programme proposals and responses to funding proposals in order to engage in needs assessments and pilot projects that will provide the illustrations and evidence to support the involvement of occupational therapy in virgin practice settings.

Future research directions

As we consider being inspired and following these new directions suggested by our changing environment, it becomes imperative that we view any innovations necessarily integrated with identified client/population need; best practice; programme development and delivery evaluation; and research. Such an approach to change provides great opportunities to move our professional knowledge base forward through understanding what, why and how we do what we do.

Research needs to be embraced as an essential component of innovation; reflection about new experiences and their value to the clients involved must become a natural element of our work. We need to become totally comfortable with the essence of qualitative inquiry to inform and enrich collection of data that will enhance our understanding of the programmes we develop as well as the assessments and interventions we pursue. This in itself will forge closer and stronger bonds between us and our clients in true partnerships.

Conclusion

It is becoming increasingly important that we, as occupational therapists, dare to venture beyond the comfortable boundaries of our well developed and expected roles. All our chapter authors have offered ideas and support for an early inculcation within student occupational therapists that will prepare them to welcome and embrace unexpected and previously untested roles and relationships with clients and families. It would appear from the students' testimonials (Chapter 4) given by Quelch, Gregory and Watanabe, that they are more than ready to accept this challenge. It would seem, however, that many practitioners may not be as ready for this shift into the unknown (Overton et al., 2009; Rodger et al, 2009); this is not surprising since changing a well-tested recipe is onerous, risky and contingent upon a clear commitment to want to try something new. Perhaps this is a good time, however, for such pioneering to be undertaken. This seems to be very similar to the beginning of occupational therapy as a profession. When rehabilitation aides were trained to help injured members of the armed forces during and after World War I, this was a time of immense challenge within the world. The aides became essential members of treatment teams in battle zones, within hospitals and convalescent facilities thus forging the first steps forward towards the exploration of the critical relationship between occupational engagement and health. The same thing could be said about today – that it is a time of immense change around a world much altered by globalisation, diasporic movement and competing political agendas. Today, societal needs for a reclaiming of a sense of community and support for human rights have become essential. The place for occupational science, occupational therapy and occupational therapists is becoming ever more clear and inviting.

References

Brown, G.T., & Rodger, S. (1999). Research utilization models: frameworks for implementing evidence-based occupational therapy practice. *Occupational Therapy International, 6* (1), 1–23.

Canadian Association of Occupational Therapists. (1991). Occupational Therapy Guidelines for Client-Centred Practice. Toronto: CAOT Publications.

Canadian Association of Occupational Therapists. (2007). Enabvling Occupation II: advancing an occupational therapy vision of health, well-being and justice through occupation. Canadian Association: Ottawa, Canada. Canadian Association of Occupational Therapists.

Carswell, A., McColl M.A., Baptiste, S, Law, M. (2004). The Canadian Occupational Performance Measure: a research and clinical literature review. *Canadian Journal of Occupational Therapy, 71* (4), 210–222.

Clark, F., Azen, S., Zemke, R., Jackson, J., Carlson, M., Mandel, D., et al. (1997). Occupational therapy for independent-living older adults. *Journal of the American Medical Association, 278* (16), 1321–1326.

Finlay, L. (1993). Nelson Thornes: London, England.

Friedland, J. (2003). Why crafts? Influences on the development of occupational therapy in Canada from 1890–1930. Muriel Driver memorial Lecture. *Canadian Journal of Occupational Therapy, 70* (4), 204–213.

Gottesfeld, H., Rhee, C., & Parker, G. (1970). A study of the role of paraprofessionals in community mental health. *Community Mental Health Journal, 6* (4), 285–291.

Jacoby, R., & Oppenheimer C. (eds). (1991). *Psychiatry in the Elderly.* Oxford: Oxford University Press.

Kronenberg, F., Algado, S., & Pollard, N. (Eds.). (2004). *Occupational Therapy Without Borders: Learning From The Spirit of Survivors.* Edinburgh: Churchill Livingstone.

Law, M., Cooper, B., Strong, S., Stewart, D., Rigby, C., Letts, L. (1993). The Person-Environment-Occupation Model: A transactive approach to occupational performance. *Canadian Journal of Occupational Therapy, 63* (1).

Leathard, A. (ed). (2003). Inter-professional Collaboration: from policy to practice in health and social care. Brunner-Routledge: East Sussex, England.

Mathiowetz, V. (1993). Role of physical performance component evaluations in occupational therapy functional assessment. *American Journal of Occupational Therapy, 47* (3), 225–230.

Ministry of Health & Long Term Care Ontario. (2010). http://www.health.gov.on.ca/transformation/fht/fht_mn.html.

Overton, A., Clark, M., Thomas, Y. (2009). A review of non-traditional occupational therapy practice palcement educatiobn: a focus on role-emerging and project placements. *British Journal of Occupational Therapy, 72* (7), 294–301.

Roger, S., Thomas, Y., Holley, S., Soringfield, E., Edwards, A., Broadbridge, J., Greber, C., McBryde, C., Banks, R., & Hawkins, R. (2009). Increasing the occupational therapy mental health workforce through innovative practice education: a pilot project. *Australian Occupational Therapy Journal, 56*, 409–417.

Sayce, L., Craig, T.K.J., & Boardman, A.P. (1991). The development of community mental health centres in the UK. *Social Psychiatry and Psychiatric Epidemiology, 26* (1), 14–20.

Townsend, E., & Polatajko, H. (Eds.). (2007). *Enabling Occupation II: Advancing an Occupational Therapy Vision for Health, Well-being, & Justice Through Occupation.* Ottawa: Canadian Association of Occupational Therapists.

Whiteford, G. (2000). Occupational deprivation: global challenge in the new millenium, *British Journal of Occupational Therapy, 63* (5), 200–204.

Wilcock, A. (1998). *An Occupational Perspective of Health.* Thorofare: Slack.

Wilcock, A. (2006). *An Occupational Perspective of Health* (2nd ed.). Thorofare: Slack.

World Health Organization (2010). International Classification of Function, Disability and Health. http://www.who.int/classifications/icf/en/. Downloaded 7 June 2010.

Index

Role Emerging Occupational Therapy: Maximising Occupation-Focused Practice, 1st edition. Edited by Miranda Thew, Mary Edwards, Sue Baptiste and Matthew Molineux. © 2011 Blackwell Publishing Ltd.